# THE
# META SHRED
# *DIET*

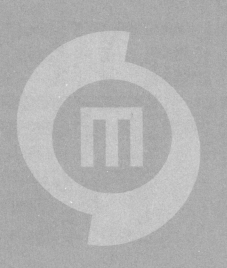

A Men'sHealth BOOK

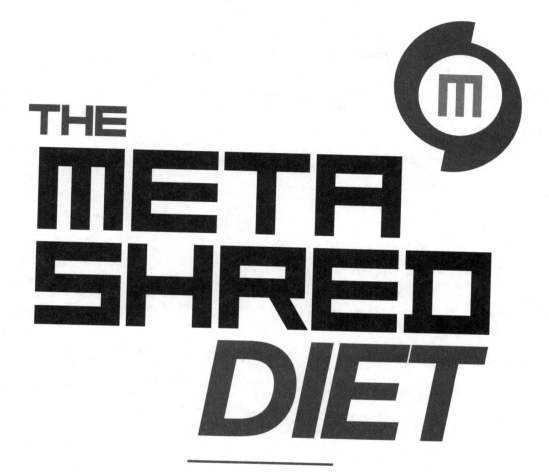

# THE META SHRED DIET

## YOUR 28-DAY RAPID FAT-LOSS PLAN.
## SIMPLE. EFFECTIVE. AMAZING.

## MICHAEL ROUSSELL, PhD

RODALE.

# RODALE wellness

*Live happy. Be healthy. Get inspired.*

Sign up today to get exclusive access to our authors, exclusive bonuses,
and the most authoritative, useful, and cutting-edge information on health, wellness,
fitness, and living your life to the fullest.

**Visit us online at RodaleWellness.com**
**Join us at RodaleWellness.com/Join**

Rodale books may be purchased for business or promotional use or for special sales.
For information, please e-mail: BookMarketing@Rodale.com.

*Men's Health*® is a registered trademark of Rodale Inc.

Printed in the United States of America

Rodale Inc. makes every effort to use acid-free ⊗, recycled paper ♻.

Photographs by Beth Bischoff

Book design by Joanna Williams

Library of Congress Cataloging-in-Publication Data is on file with the publisher.

ISBN 978-1-62336-988-0 paperback

Distributed to the trade by Macmillan

2 4 6 8 10 9 7 5 3 1

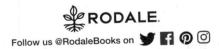

Follow us @RodaleBooks on 🐦 📘 📌 📷

We inspire health, healing, happiness, and love in the world.
Starting with you.

# Contents

# Acknowledgments

Thank you to my wife Emily Roussell. My best friend that has been with me every step of the way. You have always gone above and beyond to help and support me in my research, study, and work. I love you.

Thank you to my children Grace, Peter, David, and Joseph—you are my motivation and the life force behind what I do.

Thank you to my parents Mike and Lisa who sacrificed everything they could for decades to ensure my sisters and myself received the best education possible. I hope you find this book to be an example of quality ROI.

Thank you to my sisters Holly and Jodie for always pushing me to be as good as you both were academically and not settling for being the jock of the family. To my in-laws Jim and Sue Adams, Leo Martel, Marquis Renquin, and Charlotte Roussell: Thank you for your love and the examples that you have been for me.

I'd like to thank the many teachers, mentors, advisors, colleagues, and friends that have taken the time to talk with, teach, and invest in me: Dr. Erin Pelkey, who started me off in my journey as a scientist; Dr. Paula Tracy, who helped me see the bigger world of science and helped me follow my true passion in nutrition; Dr. Penny Kris-Etherton, who helped mentor me into a professional scientist and showed me how to look beyond conscious and unconscious biases to thoroughly analyze and review data.

I have spent a majority of my life at academic institutions and have many people to thank. From my time at St. Mark's School: Steve Bristol, Carrie Disenroth, and Jay and Whiz Hutchinson—thank you. From my time at Hobart College: Michelle Iklé, Cheryl Forbes—thank you. From my brief stint at University of Vermont Medical School: Richard

Pinckney, MD—thank you. From my time at Penn State University: John Beard, Dee Bagshaw, Amy Cifelli, and Jen Flemming—thank you.

To my many science and fitness friends and colleagues, our conversations over e-mail, at conferences, at bars after conferences, at your facilities or research labs have played a major role in the shaping and exploration of the ideas that became *The MetaShred Diet.*

Coach Dos, thank you for believing in a young kid you barely knew to write the nutrition chapter in your first (and second!) books.

Alwyn Cosgrove, thank you for always having me question my assumptions about physiology and fat loss and teaming up with me to build what was the precursor to *The MetaShred Diet* so many years ago.

Bill Hartman, I wish we spoke more because I always leave our conversations with two pages of notes. You truly appreciate the quest for becoming a modern day renaissance man.

Joe Dowdell, thank you for showing me the art of working with clients and selflessly opening so many doors for me over the years. I have the greatest respect for you.

Heather Leidy, PhD, Shalene McNeil, PhD, Chor San Khoo, PhD, Alison Hill, PhD, and Keith Scott: Thank you for your guidance and friendship.

Roy, Val, and Jubal: Thank you for believing in the true power of nutrition to impact performance in athletics and business.

To my team, Lisa Flood and Megan Colletto, RD, PhD—you are incredible to work with. I am very thankful for all your expertise, effort, and teamwork.

To all my friends and colleagues in publishing: Michael Easter, Paul Kita, Ben Court, Lou Schuler, TC Luoma, Sean Hyson, Brian Sabin, Jeff O'Connell, Abby Lerner, Brittany Risher, Amanda Jedeikin, and Cassie Shortsleeve: I appreciate your patience editing my writing and putting up with me when I missed deadlines.

Finally, to Adam Campbell: Thank you for reaching out to me as a first year graduate student to fact check some science for *Men's Health* magazine. It only took of 8 years for us to meet in person, but I appreciate our friendship and your counsel so very much. Thank you for your essential role in making this book happen.

*-Dr. Mike*

# Introduction

Recently, I caught up with a friend of mine, Jack. Like most people, Jack hadn't really changed in appearance since the last time we had seen each other, about 8 months prior. He and I made small talk for a while, hitting on topics such as our kids' obsession with Minecraft Story Mode, the increasing price of beef, and how summer TV is really bad. But as many of my conversations seem to go, Jack soon started asking me about nutrition and fat loss. It comes with the territory of being a PhD nutritionist and weight-loss advisor to *Men's Health* magazine.

Basically, Jack was pretty frustrated. He said that he had been dieting for "as long as I can remember" but, somehow, still had 15 pounds to lose. After further discussion, Jack confessed that while he was a lifetime dieter, his compliance with his fat-loss diet was pretty bad.

This resulted in a behavior that I see in a lot of people. Because Jack was supposed to be "dieting," he never felt like he could enjoy indulgent foods or foods in normal or even large quantities. He would feel guilty when he ate them, get discouraged, fall off the wagon, eat more, and then wait until Monday and start dieting again.

This cycle would repeat week after week, month after month. The upshot was that Jack wasn't losing the weight he wanted to. He was burned out and discouraged because he felt like he had been dieting forever and not getting anywhere.

Sound familiar? It happens to a lot of people. And the best cure that I've found is an all-out blitz. In fact, it's exactly why I wrote this book.

Jack was lost in the perpetual starting and stopping of 12-week fat-loss programs, so a shorter—and more extreme—program would be a better way for him to break the cycle and make a serious change. I told Jack about my 28-day rapid fat-loss program—the MetaShred Diet—and explained that there were three rules he would need to follow if he were going to do the plan.

1. **No cheating.** He needed to stick to the diet 100 percent.

2. **Complete focused effort.** No low-carb dieting and then a week later switching to Paleo, only to decide 3 days after that to try carb cycling. All of his efforts needed to be focused on losing as much fat as possible, as fast as possible.

3. **Let people know.** Telling people what he was doing would put the pressure on Jack to really make the 28-day fat-loss sprint work. In reality, 28 days isn't that long, and if he told friends and co-workers, they would be sure to check in with him to see how he was doing. (Plus, most people would assume that losing 10 to 15 pounds in 4 weeks isn't possible, so they would be intrigued enough to find out what was happening.)

He agreed that rapid fat loss was what he needed to end his lifetime of dieting. He also agreed to my three stipulations, and he started the MetaShred Diet that next Monday. And, really, that's all it takes for anyone. The rules are simple—and all you have to do is commit for 28 days.

Have you been dieting forever?

If so, you're not alone. I have yet to meet with a client for the first time who has never lost weight. They have all lost weight. The problem is that they all just regained the weight or stalled out with their weight loss.

They felt trapped in this mind-set that they *should* be dieting. So any and all social situations where "forbidden foods" were served were accompanied with guilt and plenty of remorseful thoughts, such as, "I probably shouldn't have had that [insert decadent food or drink]."

Let me tell you: I have no time or tolerance for food guilt. And neither should you. Life is too short.

Nutrition is so powerful because you are only one meal away from moving in the right direction. Your next meal—whether it's breakfast, lunch, or dinner—is your opportunity to say with your actions, *I'm making a change now. Moving forward, it's going to be different.*

The time to end a lifetime of dieting is now, and you deserve to be in the best shape of your life.

Let's make that happen together.

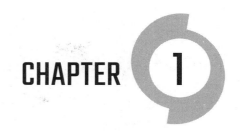

## CHAPTER 1

# Get the Results You Really Want

Experts generally talk about weight loss as if it is one thing: the act of burning off body fat to reduce total body weight. As a result, lots of cookie-cutter weight-loss programs are developed and eventually fail. This is partly due to the fact that weight loss is not one thing.

There are two kinds of weight loss: rapid weight loss and long-term weight loss. Neglecting the differences between these two kinds of weight loss is a recipe for disaster. Here's why: If you wanted to be a great sprinter, would you hire a world-renowned marathon coach? No.

So if you wanted to lose 15 pounds in the next 28 days, does it make sense to follow a plan designed to help you lose weight over a period of 6 months? No.

Rapid fat loss and long-term weight loss requires a different mind-set, different actions, and a different approach to manipulating and dealing with your biochemistry. One is not better than the other, but it all depends on what you want to accomplish and the timeline to which you want to adhere.

The MetaShred Diet is a rapid fat-loss program. Everything about it, from the mind-set you need to adopt to how you will manipulate your carbohydrate intake to how you will approach sleeping, is tailored to helping you peel off as much body fat as possible in 28 days.

# Permission Granted: Don't Be Realistic

I once had a client, Tom, lose 21 pounds in 28 days. At one point, he was averaging a weight loss of 1 pound per day! That's exceptional, but it's exactly what he was planning to do. Seriously, his goal was to lose 21 pounds in 28 days. Yes, it was aggressive, but he believed he could do it, and we structured an effective science-based plan to get him there. The plan he used was generation one of the MetaShred Diet.

I bring up Tom's success to emphasize that we need to get aggressive with our goals for this program. There is a slow-growing movement that we need to be realistic with our weight-loss goals and avoid setting our expectations too high. On the surface, this seems like good advice: Set realistic weight-loss goals so that you don't get frustrated and quit, as you would likely do if you didn't reach your unrealistic goals.

But what does science say? Are smaller, more realistic goals motivating because they are easier to achieve, or are more audacious goals the way to go because you are motivated to achieve something great and so different than your current state?

When it comes to weight loss, how realistic your goals are may have little impact on the amount of weight that you lose. And intentionally being conservative may actually hurt your results. In a University of Minnesota weight-loss study, researchers found that, on average, participants' goals were 24 percent too high. Yet those who tried to lose 16 percent of their body weight—instead of the commonly recommended 5 to 10 percent[1]— dropped more pounds than their conservative counterparts. The scientists speculated that those who set more aggressive goals understand that it takes more effort to lose more weight.

So when you set an audacious weight-loss goal, you know that it will require more effort, and that effort will reap a greater reward. In the end, effort is all we can control, so anything that increases your drive to put forth more effort will give you greater weight loss.

# Focus on Action Goals

Big audacious weight-loss goals are the way to go for the MetaShred Diet, because you need total commitment during these 28 days. But spending time dreaming about being 15 pounds lighter in less than a month isn't 100 percent productive—it's more like zero percent productive. The downside of large and aggressive goals is that they can seem so unrealistic that you aren't sure where to start, you get overwhelmed, and you don't attack your plan.

This is why I'm going to ask you to set two kinds of goals. The first is the big, aggressive, audacious goal. You'll never lose 15 pounds in 28 days if you don't expect to. People tend to rise to their levels of expectation, so expect a lot from yourself. That's the big-picture stuff. This is your end-point goal.

On the micro, day-to-day level, I want you to be practical and realistic. You aren't going to lose 15 pounds in 1 day, so don't act like you need to. On a day-to-day basis, you need to be methodical, realistic, and logistics-focused.

Your daily goal list should include things like:

- I will complete a 30-minute workout.
- I will eat my three MetaShred meals.
- I will go to bed with the lights out by 10:30 p.m.

These are your action goals. They are the *realistic* action-oriented goals achieved day in and day out that will allow you to lose the weight you want. What's more, University of Iowa researchers found that people are more likely to stick with their weight-loss plans when they concentrate on specific *actions* instead of the desired result. The likely reason: This allows you to realize success even before it shows up on the scale or in the mirror, which helps keep you motivated.[2]

Your action goals get you moving every day, working toward your end-point goal.

Setting these two kinds of goals is essential if you want to get the most out of the MetaShred Diet.

## Launch an All-Out Attack

My colleague and fellow *Men's Health* magazine advisor Alwyn Cosgrove, a top expert in the fitness industry, once told me about a conversation he had with a new client about goals and expectations. She informed Alwyn that she wanted to "exercise as little as possible, eat as bad as possible, and look as good as possible."

If we're being honest with ourselves, this is how most of us view healthy living. We want to live as healthy as we need to stay fit and free of chronic disease, but not much past that. This is why much of the work that I do with my private clients focuses on modifying and improving their current behaviors, so that, over time, the changes will yield improvements in health and facilitate weight loss. I help clients "hack" their current habits so that they get better results doing essentially what they're already doing. This approach works, but it's slow. That's the trade-off.

The MetaShred Diet is *not* about hacking habits to get you better results over time. The MetaShred Diet is about getting after it. It is an all-out war on your adipocytes. (That's sciencespeak for your fat cells.) It is an all-out war on your environment, which is trying to coax you into eating more carbs and calories while also discouraging you from exercising or even just moving around. (Yes, your environment is out to make you fail; we'll talk about how to fix that later.)

This mind-set shift away from gradual adjustments to an all-out and aggressive upgrade of your diet and metabolism is essential to having massive success with the MetaShred Diet.

The doughnuts are always warm. You can order Domino's pizza with your voice via Amazon Echo. Your couch is always calling with your favorite show. You are always in enemy territory. Act accordingly.

# Create Your Own Research Study

One of the reasons that the MetaShred Diet works so well is that it is grounded in decades of research on nutrition, metabolism, and weight loss. Aside from the scientific foundation, the other hallmark difference between the MetaShred Diet and any other rapid fat-loss plan available to you is the intensified synergistic effort of the components of the diet.

We aren't throwing out all of the effective strategies that science has uncovered for long-term weight loss; we're just intensifying them in order to squeeze out all of their fat-burning ability in a 28-day period instead of a 6-month period.

Consider a nutrition study that can give you a direct cause-and-effect relationship between the food or diet being studied and a specific outcome is called a controlled feeding study. This is the kind of study that I ran at Pennsylvania State University as a graduate student. In this kind of study, all of the foods and beverages are weighed and measured with precision and then given to each individual to eat. Study participants aren't supposed to consume anything outside of what's given to them, except for water, tea, and coffee.

If this sounds intense, that's because it is intense! It also gets results. Customized, data-driven diets work. That's exactly what I've created for you with the MetaShred Diet. I'll show you how to easily determine which MetaDiet Level is right for you (starting on page 194) so that you can follow a customized meal plan to get the results you want. You are your own research project, and I am your lab assistant, here to make sure that everything works as you need it to.

If you have any questions along the way, just hit me up on Twitter @mikeroussell and use the hashtag #metashred

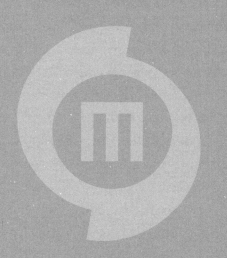

## CHAPTER 2

# Why This Diet Is Different— And Why It Has to Be

For decades, the math of fat loss was presented as a very simple and straightforward calculation. All you needed to do was use an equation to determine how many calories a person was burning each day and then create a diet that provides fewer calories than that.

At the most basic level, weight loss is achieved when calories in (CI) are exceeded by calories out (CO). Thus . . .

**calories in < calories out = weight loss!**

Existing, eating, digesting, thinking, moving, shopping, working, and all your other daily activities require energy. Your body needs to get that energy from somewhere. The main source of energy for your body is the food you eat.

When you don't provide your body with enough energy through food, it then goes to its energy reserves—you know this as body fat—to get the energy it needs. One of the first nutrition and obesity courses I took in college painted this very clear picture of weight loss. The instructor said that getting into this needed energy deficit was as simple as "reducing calorie intake by 500 to 1,000 calories per day."

That sounds simple, but it's not effective.

I deem this rationale for achieving weight loss as ineffective because it has not actually simplified, but instead diluted, the fat-loss road map. Nutrition and health students all over the world are taught to reduce someone's calorie intake somewhere between 500 and 1,000 calories per day to elicit weight loss of 1 to 2 pounds per week.

Here's the diluted rationale behind this:

- 1 pound of fat contains 3,500 calories
- 3,500 calories/7 days = 500 calories/day

- 2 pounds of fat contains 7,000 calories
- 7,000 calories/7 days = 1,000 calories/day

If you consume 500 to 1,000 calories less per day, you will create an energy deficit of 500 to 1,000 calories per day, which will create a weekly energy deficit of 3,500 to 7,000 calories. That equates to losing 1 to 2 pounds of fat per week.

It's so logical that it sounds like it should work, right? Unfortunately, weight loss isn't that simple. If it was, you wouldn't be reading this book—since you could have just cut 500 calories a day from your diet and, by the end of a year, lost 52 pounds of fat!

One of the issues with this flawed fat-loss logic that is force-fed to students (and to you) via textbooks and uninformed health professionals is that it doesn't consider the ongoing complex system of checks and balances that are in your body.

Here's a simple example: When you reduce the calories that you're eating by 500 per day, your body automatically stops burning as many calories as it had been previously. Remember how your body needs calories for existing, eating, digesting, thinking, moving, shopping, and working? Let's say that it takes your body 2,000 calories to do all those things. Once you reduce how many calories you're eating, your body senses this and responds by becoming more efficient. The impact: It will now only take 1,800 calories to exist, eat, digest, think, move, shop, and work. So instead of having a calorie deficit of 500 calories per day, you actually only have a deficit of 300 calories per day.

The other problem with the calories in < calories out approach to weight loss is that it doesn't take into account how different foods behave in your body. All foods and calories are viewed as the same. Thus, creating an energy deficit by eating 500 calories less of protein compared to 500 calories less of sugar is seen as the same thing.

If you think that sounds crazy, you're right. So much so that the lunacy of the all-calories-are-created-equal mind-set gave rise to the Carbohydrate-Insulin Hypothesis.

## The Carbohydrate-Insulin Hypothesis

Because the calories in < calories out approach didn't seem to be as effective at helping people lose weight as most would have hoped, some scientists set off to find a more elegant biochemical-based explanation for weight gain and weight loss. The result was the Carbohydrate-Insulin Hypothesis (CIH).

To best understand the CIH, it's important to first discuss how carbohydrates and the hormone insulin interact in your body. When you eat carbohydrates, your body breaks those carbohydrates down into glucose—the simplest form of sugar—and dumps it into your bloodstream. This causes the sugar, or glucose, levels in your blood to rise.

Your body senses this rise in sugar and signals your pancreas to release the hormone insulin. Insulin's primary job is to help maintain blood sugar in an optimal range. It does this by shuttling excess sugar out of your bloodstream and into your muscles and fat cells.

Sometimes, if you eat a lot of carbohydrates, your pancreas gets a little "trigger happy" and overshoots the amount of insulin needed, resulting in too much sugar being removed from your bloodstream.

Have you ever had a large, usually refined, carbohydrate meal only to find yourself hungry an hour or so later? This is a result of a trigger-happy pancreas that released too much insulin and subsequently drove your blood sugar too low. When your blood sugar is low, your body releases signals that spur you to eat, in order to correct the blood sugar imbalance.

You might be wondering, in this situation, if your body just stuffed a bunch of sugar into fat and muscle cells, why doesn't it just let some of it back into the bloodstream?

Great question. For your muscles, sugar is a one-way street. Sugar goes in, but your muscles don't have the cellular roadways to let it back out again. The only option is for your muscles to use the sugar to fuel your muscle contractions.

Your fat cells *can* give back energy to your body, but it's in the form of fat—not sugar—and it won't do this when your insulin levels are high. You might say that your body doesn't like to waste effort. As a result, your cells can't take in energy (sugar going into fat cells) and give out energy (fat being released from fat cells) at the same time. In fact, insulin blocks your fat cells from releasing energy.

What we are stuck with here is the crux of the CIH.

- High levels of insulin stuffing fat cells with sugar
- Low levels of blood sugar due to the "overshooting" of insulin

- High levels of hunger—due to low blood sugar—along with insulin blocking your fat cells from releasing energy

The end result is that people eat more because their bodies are telling them that they are hungry, even though technically, there is an abundance of energy trapped in their fat cells. This process is intensified when you consider the fact that as we gain weight, our bodies become less sensitive to insulin.

Here's a simple example to illustrate what happens when you have decreased insulin sensitivity (also known as being insulin resistant). Let's say you eat a bowl of pasta and your blood sugar increases from 100 points to 125 points. If your body releases five units of insulin, that is enough to get your blood sugar back down to 100 points.

Now, imagine yourself 20 pounds heavier. You eat the same bowl of pasta, your blood sugar goes from 100 points to 125 points, but when your body releases 5 units of insulin, your blood sugar only goes down to 110 points. Weight gain—and stress, sleep deprivation, and being sedentary—makes your body less sensitive to insulin. Your body then releases another 5 or 10 units of insulin in an effort to finally get your blood sugar back to 100 points.

The state of being insulin resistant means that your body will be releasing above-normal levels of insulin which, per the CIH, will only sustain the lockdown of energy in your fat cells, while driving hunger even more. The solution to obesity is to control insulin by eating fewer carbohydrates. Less insulin then frees your fat cells to release as much energy as they want, allowing you to lose weight.

It's quite a compelling story. It gets better when many proponents of the CIH state that you are "hormonally optimized" for fat loss by controlling insulin. You can eat as much as you want, as hormonal optimization trumps calorie counting.

Don't you love it when you're told that you can eat as much as you want and still lose weight? Who wouldn't want to do that? The CIH for weight loss is very appealing to people because it contains all of the key components to a great diet story.

1. **It's not your fault.** If you haven't lost weight in the past, it's because you were given bad advice. The rationale behind calories in < calories out are flawed and not robust enough scientifically.

2. **It's based on hard-core science**. The CIH delves into the complicated science of hormonal responses to food and hormonal regulation of fat cells. Something so scientific has to be true, right?

3. **It gives you permission to indulge.** As long as a food doesn't raise insulin levels, the CIH allows you to eat as much of it as you want. For example, you can eat butter! As much as you want!

The CIH tells you what you want to hear. It highlights the importance of the hormonal effects of the foods that we eat, but it doesn't solve the entire weight-loss puzzle—and weight-loss research has not yielded universal support. From a practical standpoint, I've never had any luck helping a client lose weight when I tell them that they can eat as much as they want.

## Where Does That Leave You?

When formulating the MetaShred Diet, I set out to compile for you the most effective fat-loss program that you could get your hands on. To do this, I didn't discount and disregard the calories in < calories out approach or Carbohydrate-Insulin Hypothesis for weight loss, but instead fused together the best parts of both methodologies.

By controlling calories and selecting the types of calories that create an optimal hormonal environment to burn fat, we can take the brakes off of your fat loss and deliver the rapid results that you've been in search of.

## Rapid Weight-Loss Scams

Type "rapid weight loss" into the search engine of your choice, and you'll be overwhelmed with the more than 18 million search results promising a variety of foods, diets, and cures to reach that goal.

Next, head over to Amazon and look at the top three weight-loss supplements. The first two products feature compounds that science has literally shown do not lead to weight loss in humans, while the third product has been shunned by thousands of people due to the horrible digestive side effects. (But side effects aside, it won't speed weight loss.)

Now, turn on the TV to find an afternoon talk show touting a 2-week rapid weight-loss diet that promises to remove the foods making you sick, while providing you a list of foods that you can eat as much of as you want.

Two quick points about these specific promises: First, if a food is making you sick, then it has probably been laced with *E. coli*. Aside from food allergies (which are impossible to mass diagnose via an afternoon talk show), no food induces weight-loss-zapping illness. Second, if a book, article, TV show, or expert ever promises you a list of foods that you can eat unlimited amounts of, close the browser tab, close the book, change the channel, or get up and walk away. You can never—and I rarely use the word "never"—eat as much of anything as you want. You can't even drink unlimited amounts of water.

Finally, click on any superfood rapid weight-loss article on Facebook, and you'll quickly discover that the foods discussed do not elicit rapid weight loss, or weight loss at all. More likely this was just a compelling title used to entice you to check out the story (a.k.a. clickbait!).

When you distill down the "rapid weight-loss solutions" available today, there are three recurring themes. Let's look at each and why they aren't going to help you at all.

## Scam #1: The Cleanse

Here's the big promise: Your body is overloaded with toxins that have accumulated through the strain of modern living. These toxins are causing your body to hold on to fat, and they are causing your fat cells to get jammed up, as if they were in a metabolic grid-lock. If you cleanse your system, the toxins will be released, and your fat cells will then be free to release all of their pent-up fat. As a result, the weight will melt right off. Good story, right?

Total fantasy.

But, you might say, when people go on these cleanses, they do lose weight. So there must be some truth to them, right? There isn't. Whether it's the original cheap cleanse—requiring you to down a cocktail of lemon juice, maple syrup, and cayenne pepper several times a day—or today's more high-brow juice cleanse, which asks you to fork over serious cash for essentially sugar water that has been rebranded as cold-pressed juice (made from handpicked organic fruits and vegetables), the sad truth is this: It's really just extreme calorie restriction that causes the weight loss.

There is no such thing as a diet cleanse. You don't need to cleanse anything. That's why you have a liver. These methods don't cause you to lose weight because you are "detoxing" your system. They yield weight loss because you are *starving* your system. You lose muscle; you lose fat; you lose water. So, in the end, the scale shows a lower number.

But there is nothing safe and effective about prolonged deprivation. Let's all agree to stop with the cleansing.

## Scam #2: "Medical" Weight Loss

Medical weight loss sounds very official, as if it is a really effective special weight-loss strategy that the medical community has developed as *the* solution for getting people to lose a lot of weight quickly. Unfortunately, it isn't. This term almost always refers to a method that's brute force weight loss at its worst: severe calorie restriction. The plan is usually executed via prepackaged shakes or smoothies that provide you with such a small amount of calories that it would be irresponsible *not* to have a physician overseeing what you are doing. That's because you're toeing the line between dieting and complete deprivation.

In weight-loss research, this approach is called a very low calorie diet, or VLCD. The National Institute of Diabetes and Digestive and Kidney Diseases defines VLCDs this way: "A special diet that provides up to 800 calories per day. VLCDs use commercial formulas, usually liquid shakes, soups, or bars, which replace all of your regular meals."[1] They provide a moderate amount of protein—in a weak effort to prevent total decimation of your muscle mass—a relatively high amount of carbohydrates, and a very small amount of fat. VLCDs ignore everything about the hormonal effects of weight loss and rely solely on the calories in < calories out approach—taken to the extreme.

Despite the methodology being decades old, in my travels as a nutrition educator for medical professionals, I still speak with physicians around the country who see VLCDs as the *only* way for people to lose a significant amount of weight. A VLCD may allow you to lose weight quickly, but you are almost guaranteed to put it back on.

## Scam #3: Diuretics

How is this still a thing? The use of diuretics for rapid weight loss is strangely still used by people wanting to lose weight and by people at the latter stages of weight loss who are trying to get ripped. In either case, don't waste your time.

The idea is that diuretics help you excrete excess water from your body, which leads to quick weight loss and reveals increased muscle definition. But I have helped professional fighters make weight for fights and fitness models get shredded for photo shoots—both with and without diuretics—and there is never that much of a difference. If anything, the use of diuretics further promotes dehydration, which makes you feel and perform worse.

Diuretics are formulated in many ways, but the most common ingredients that you'll see are caffeine, dandelion, and uva ursi. Caffeine is actually not a diuretic. Research shows that it can contribute to increased urination for the first couple of hours after consumption—in people who don't consume caffeine—but that's it. It doesn't seem to impact your body's fluid balance when you look at the entire day.

Despite the popularity of dandelion extract as a major component for diuretic supplements, the scientific evidence is essentially nonexistent. Dandelions are very high in potassium, making them a nice addition to a salad. But a dandelion supplement is rather useless.

Uva ursi, also known as bearberry, has been used in traditional medicine practices for centuries. As with dandelion, there is no good scientific evidence to give us a glimmer of hope that it would help as a diuretic, let alone with weight loss. But unlike dandelion extract, uva ursi has the added danger of being toxic to your liver.

In reality, your kidneys are the true regulators of fluid balance in your body. Even without the help of supplements or drugs, they have the ability to leave you up or down 4 pounds on any given day, depending on your body size and what you've had to eat. Drastically increasing carbohydrates and/or sodium can lead to increased water retention. That's why one of the strongest diuretic effects that you can elicit in your body is achieved by simply going on a carbohydrate-restricted diet, like the MetaShred Diet.

When you cut carbs, insulin is not there to signal your kidneys to retain sodium, so your kidneys excrete more water than normal. You can experience this as drastic weight loss in the first 24 to 48 hours.

But the bottom line on supplemental diuretics is this: They won't speed your ability to actually lose fat. So don't waste your money.

## Take the Brakes Off Your Fat Loss

Let's clear the air here about rapid weight loss. There is *zero* scientific data available to qualify that any rate of fat loss is unhealthy. Read that again. There is no such thing as a rate of weight loss that is unhealthy or dangerous.

The health and medical communities seems to have fallen in love with the concept of safely losing 1 to 2 pounds per week. This has been repeated so many times that people take it as a scientifically validated fact and that losing anything beyond that is unsafe. I've actually had clients come to me because their physician was concerned that they were losing weight too fast (3 pounds per week) with their new nutrition and exercise program. The doctor was worried about the health ramifications. But what about the health ramifications of keeping the fat on?

Let's demystify the supposition that safe and healthy weight loss equates to 1 to 2 pounds per week. The origin of this safe weight-loss range ties directly into the calories in < calories out belief system. Earlier in this chapter, I took you through the logic of this approach, where subtracting 500 to 1,000 calories per day would yield 1 to 2 pounds of weight loss per week. The idea being that it's not safe for a person to subtract more than 1,000 calories per day from his or her diet. This is true if you were only eating, say, 1,500 calories a day. That's because it would increase your likelihood of nutrient inadequacy and potentially lead to malnutrition. But what if you were eating 4,000 calories a day? You could cut your calories by 2,000 a day and still be eating in a healthy manner. What's more, you could increase your activity, which boosts your calorie burn and helps you lose weight even faster.

Many people are surprised to know the origin of these numbers. They're not from a collection of clinical trials looking at weight-loss rates and health outcomes, but instead a basic arithmetic exercise that doesn't account for a person's individual calorie intake, current body weight, or activity level.

Ultimately, the basis for only losing 1 to 2 pounds a week as a weight-loss benchmark isn't relevant to you, as it's a broad recommendation that's completely arbitrary. So the question is: What are you capable of? Three pounds per week? Four pounds per week?

Here's where I want your head to be when it comes to weight loss: You have no idea what you are capable of. I have no idea what you are capable of. As former Navy SEAL David Goggins says, "When you think you have given everything, you are at around 40 percent of your maximum effort."[2] With the MetaShred Diet, I want to help you break through and access that other 60 percent of your fat-loss potential.

This program is built on a collection of scientific principles that I have road tested to ensure maximum results. But everyone's maximum rate of weight loss is different. You might currently weigh 215 pounds and your goal weight is 150 pounds. Losing 5 pounds per week wouldn't be out of the ordinary. Or you might currently weigh 125 pounds and your goal weight is 120 pounds. Losing 1 pound per week will require a lot of effort. My point: Don't get hung up on the numbers. Work hard, stick to the plan, adjust as needed, and, when the fat starts peeling off, lean into it and double down on your efforts.

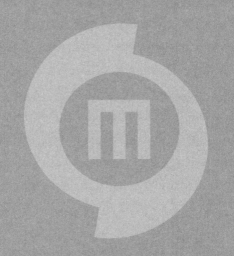

## CHAPTER 3

# Big Metabolism Lies

Just as you've been lied to regarding rapid weight loss, you've also been lied to about your metabolism. Don't feel bad: We've all been lied to. In fact, when I go over the science that debunks these metabolism myths in my seminars, I shock everyone, from registered dietitians to fitness professionals.

Before I delve into these big metabolism lies, it's important to quickly review what your metabolism is and how your body burns calories. *Metabolism* is a word used to sum up the process that your body goes through to turn food and drinks into energy. Functionally, this is the number of calories that you burn each day, also known as your total energy expenditure (TEE). Your TEE is the sum of a few different components: basal metabolic rate (BMR), the thermic effect of food (TEF), and calories burned from activity. The calories that you burn from activity can be further broken down into deliberate exercise—running, weight lifting, playing basketball—and nonexercise activity thermogenesis (NEAT). (See "Metabolism 101" on page 20.)

A major focus for fat loss is revving up your metabolic engine. But it is this search for novel ways to burn more calories throughout the day that has led to some of the most pervasive myths in all of weight loss. Here are three of the biggest.

## Lie #1: You Can Just Run It Off

Need to lose weight? Just do more exercise. *If I can just run more or work out longer, I'll be able to lose more fat faster.* This is a thought process that we are all guilty of entertaining or acting on at one time or another. I have seen it with clients, from people with regular jobs all the way up to professional athletes.

It seems like it should make sense, because we have all been taught to believe that the additive theory of energy expenditure is how our bodies function. The additive theory of energy expenditure states that, with increasing amounts of activity, calories burned from

# METABOLISM 101

Here are some basic terms related to metabolism that you should be familiar with.

**Calorie:** A calorie is the unit of measurement that we use to describe the amount of energy contained in food.

**Basal metabolic rate (BMR):** You may also hear the term resting energy expenditure (REE). While there are slight scientific differences between REE and BMR, for our purposes, they are the same thing. Both are a measurement of the number of calories that your body burns at rest. Essentially, this is how many calories that your body would need to sustain itself if you laid in bed all day long.

**Thermic effect of food (TEF):** It takes energy for your body to extract energy from the food you eat. Digesting, breaking down, and metabolizing a steak takes work! The calories that your body expends during this process is known as the thermic effect of food. Different nutrients take different amounts of

energy to process. This was initially quantified by scientists in the 1920s, when they discovered that people's metabolic rates increased after they ate certain foods. Protein has the greatest thermic effect and can cause about a 20 to 30 percent increase in metabolism. Carbohydrates can increase metabolism by 5 to 10 percent, while fat has essentially no impact on metabolic rate.[1]

**Nonexercise activity thermogenesis (NEAT):** This is just a fancy term to describe the calories that you burn from activities such as walking from the parking lot to your office, washing your car, and even fidgeting at your desk. Basically, as the name suggests, it accounts for the extra calories burned through activity that's not deliberate exercise.

**Total energy expenditure (TEE):** This number reflects the total amount of calories that you burn on a daily basis. It includes calories burned from your basal metabolic rate and all daily activities.

those activities are simply added together, and that, with more exercise, more calories are burned in a linear fashion.

The problem with this line of thinking is that it doesn't fit the survival-of-the-fittest model of biology. When it comes to understanding how systems in our bodies work, it has always benefited me to think about how a particular process would help someone survive. If the process would help a human survive, then it's probably how the body works.

This additive model of calorie burning fails the survival-of-the-fittest test miserably. If you were a lone hunter-gatherer, and you had to travel 5, 10, or 25 miles in a day to find food, it wouldn't bode well for you if your body continued to burn more and more calories without any adjustments to your metabolism. Imagine that you did indeed have to travel 25 miles—you'd expend about 2,500 calories. (Humans typically burn about 100 calories per mile.) But now suppose a hunter-gatherer friend of yours only burned 1,000 calories to go 25 miles. Who would have the better chance of survival? Your friend would, since his body began to conserve energy as his physical activity increased. The total amount of calories that he burned was constrained, irrespective of his doing more and more activity.

This is the constrained theory of total energy expenditure, and it more accurately explains how our bodies burn calories and why you can't just run off all the extra pounds. With the constrained theory of total energy expenditure, your body downregulates its calorie-burning processes. For example, your organs expend less energy, and your muscles become more efficient so that they can do the same amount of work, but burn fewer calories doing so. At the most basic level, these are all protective measures by the body to ensure survival.

Humans are not the only ones to do this. When you look at the energy expenditures of different species, like rodents or birds, they all follow this constrained model for expending energy.

Back in 1992, Klaas R. Westerterp, PhD, and his colleagues in the Department of Human Biology at University of Limburg in the Netherlands, conducted a 40-week study that clearly illustrated how the body conserves energy when energy output becomes too high. In this study, they recruited 23 nonexercising men and women to undergo 40 weeks of half-marathon training. The study participants ran four times per week and increased their running times from 10 minutes up to 90 minutes over the course of the study. Despite the increase in calorie-burning from their new running regimen, the people in the study tried to keep the amount of food they were eating the same. Almost right off the bat, both men and women in the study experienced an increase in the total amount of calories that they were burning daily.[2]

However, these increases in total calorie-burning slowed almost as fast as they started to increase. Thanks to a thoughtful analysis by Herman Pontzer, PhD, an associate professor of anthropology at Hunter College in Manhattan, beyond 20 minutes of running, the study participants started to conserve energy and not burn as many calories as predicted. If they exercised longer, they didn't actually burn more calories, as would be assumed. It seems that significantly increasing the amount of exercise, without modifying what they were eating, takes the body out of what I call the metabolic sweet spot.

The work by Dr. Westerterp and the additional analysis by Dr. Pontzer show us that the body hates the idea of "running it off" just as much as you do. You need a more sophisticated approach that optimizes the relationship between what you are eating and how much you are burning, so that you can maximize the effect you get from the exercise. This is what I set out to do when I designed the MetaShred Diet.

## Lie #2: Cheat Meals Boost Your Metabolism

In 1974, in his commencement address to graduates of California Institute of Technology, theoretical physicist Richard P. Feynman, PhD, told the students, "The first principle is that you must not fool yourself—and you are the easiest person to fool."[3] This Nobel laureate in physics probably didn't realize that he was also giving the graduating class some of the best weight-loss advice they would ever receive.

The lore of gorging yourself on a cheat meal to increase your metabolism has become pervasive in dieting circles, because we have been able to convince ourselves of the greatest con ever: Overeating is good for weight loss.

Trust me, it isn't. Or don't trust me: I'll just show you the data.

There are people you may know or have read about who maintain low body fat percentages and regularly indulge in daylong cupcake-fueled benders. But, for every one of those people you know, I could show you five people who only allow themselves 5 to 6 cheat days per year in order to maintain single-digit body fat levels 24/7/365.

The truth is—and you know this at a logical, nonemotional level—overeating or *cheating* isn't going to enhance the rate of your fat loss.

The big promise—and every lie needs a big promise—with overeating/cheating to enhance fat loss is that this strategy *fixes* the decrease in your metabolic rate that normally occurs with dieting. In 2006, researchers from the Mayo Clinic wanted to look at the effects of overeating on people's metabolic rates. Instead of looking at just one meal, they looked at consecutive weeks of overeating. But we just need to look at the results at the end of Week 1. In this study, James A. Levine, MD, PhD, and his colleagues overfed 16 study participants by 1,000 calories per day ("Honey, I have to eat these two extra slices of pizza in the name of science!"). After 7 days of overeating, the average metabolic rate increased by 18 calories.[4] You read that right: 18 calories. You don't need your PhD to realize that the fat-loss math doesn't add up if you need to overeat by 1,000 calories to burn an extra 18.

Most people aren't going to overeat for a whole week while dieting, although I've seen people employ this approach in the middle of their diets to give their bodies "a break and fix their metabolisms." The data speaks for itself here.

But what about a more traditional cheat? The good old cheat day. One day of gluttony in hopes of metabolic glory. Does it work? I'm assuming you can guess the answer to this question by now, but let's take a look at what the data says. At the University of Lausanne in Switzerland, researchers gave people an extra 700 calories from bread, rice, biscuits, and sugar.[5] What did these dedicated carb overeaters get for their efforts? No increase in basal metabolic rate, but a 7 percent increase in 24-hour energy expenditure. Seven percent! That sounds great, as percentages often do. But unfortunately, this only translates to an extra 138 calories burned. The researchers attributed 35 of these calories to being "calories needed to metabolize and process the additional food," or the thermic effect of food.

The researchers weren't sure what the cause of the additional calories expended actually was. Since the study participants' basal metabolic rates didn't increase, the most probable explanation was that it was due to an increase in NEAT. I'm pretty confident that you can just move more and take an extra 2,000 to 3,000 steps during the day to increase your NEAT by 100 calories, without needing to eat an extra 700 calories.

We have just looked at two overfeeding studies, but there are a lot of them, and the bottom line is always the same: You never end up burning more calories than you consume, and the increases in your metabolic rate or fat-burning hormones are transient, at best, and never enough to have a noticeable positive effect.

Whenever you feel the urge to *boost* your metabolism with a double bacon cheeseburger in the midst of the MetaShred Diet, just remember the sage words of Dr. Feynman.

## Lie #3: Eating More Frequently Boosts Your Metabolism

This big metabolism lie has bamboozled people—myself included!—for decades: Eating more frequently increases your metabolism and is essential for fat loss. What's so interesting about this metabolism lie is how dogmatic it became with zero scientific support. With the other two myths we debunked, there were trails of potential scientific evidence dating back multiple decades, but this one? It's 100 percent "broscience."

The origins of increasing the frequency of your meals to increase your metabolism truly comes from the bros: bodybuilders. For decades, bodybuilders have consumed massive amounts of food seemingly nonstop throughout the day. Even in the bodybuilding cult classic movie *Pumping Iron*—which chronicles the success of Arnold Schwarzenegger's bodybuilding career—there is video footage of Arnold and his bodybuilding buddies eating what looks like all of the protein that was in the kitchen of a local restaurant.

The logic (or illogic) here is simple. Bodybuilders eat six to eight times throughout the day. Bodybuilders have high metabolisms and low body fat. Thus, eating six to eight times per day increases metabolism, which leads to low body fat. As a result, every person who steps foot out of the cubicle and into a gym needs to start eating eight times per day in order to rev up their metabolism and get lean.

This is a great example of correlation but not causation. Bodybuilders eat six to eight times a day and have high metabolisms, but eating six to eight times per day does not cause their high metabolisms.

Instead, here is the more likely scenario. Bodybuilders train with weights very frequently (five to seven times per week) and for long durations (1 to 2 hours), with the goal of getting big muscles. This results in a very high energy expenditure. And because they want to *gain* muscle mass, they must eat more calories than they are burning on a daily basis. This means that they need to eat a lot of food.

If you've ever tried to eat a lot of food consistently, you know that there is a limit to how much you can eat at one sitting. So it's easier to eat more often—hence the 6 to 8 meals per day that bodybuilders traditionally consume. Plus, the more muscle a bodybuilder gains, the more calories he will burn, leading to the need to eat even *more* to stay in a caloric surplus for muscle-building. This is why some of the biggest bodybuilders will literally eat upward of 10 times per day.

But let's take this a step further, just in case you find yourself in a Facebook debate with a certified "broscientist." The only plausible way that eating more often could increase your metabolism would be if it resulted in a greater thermic effect of food compared to eating less frequently. If the act of simply initiating and carrying out the process of digestion requires additional energy, then the more times during the day that you could do it, the greater your calorie burn would be.

Unfortunately, how you break up your meals during the day doesn't seem to have an impact on your overall number of calories burned. There just isn't any good scientific data to support the idea that the thermic effect of food over a 24-hour period is different if you eat all of your food in one meal versus dividing that same food between six meals. Eating more often as a means of revving up your metabolism is really the poster child for broscience.

In fact, when non-bodybuilders try to adopt bodybuilding habits into their lives, it rarely works out for the best. If you've ever tried to train like a bodybuilder, lifting weights 6 days a week, in addition to doing 60 minutes of cardio each day, you know what I mean. Likewise, eating like a bodybuilder comes with its own issues, specifically the two that follow.

**1. You could be more likely to overeat.** The more often you eat, the more opportunities you have for overeating. In Chapter 5, we'll discuss sleep and the impacts of inadequate sleep on weight gain/loss. However, one of the thoughts behind lack of sleep and weight gain is that when you sleep less, you are up more, giving yourself more opportunities to eat. It's the same here: The more times you eat, the more chances you have to overeat.

**2. You may adopt obsessive behaviors.** Bodybuilders are a committed breed of people who generally put bodybuilding-driven eating and training ahead of everything else. This is probably not you, so if you tried to eat six to eight times each day, you would run into some problems. For instance, I've had clients share stories of getting in trouble at work for taking too many breaks to eat. They felt as if they had to in order to lose the weight they wanted. They didn't have to and don't have to . . . and neither do you.

Keep in mind, I'm not saying that the way a professional bodybuilder eats is wrong. I'm saying that it's likely wrong for *you*.

## A Modern Approach to an Old Problem

My point in busting all of these metabolism myths isn't to criticize other programs. It's to show you, with actual science, that many of the eating rules you may have learned over the years are unnecessary. My intent is to help you focus on the details that truly matter, and in a way that easily fits *your* life—all to give you the simplest formula possible for losing fat rapidly. And I'll show you that exact formula in the next chapter.

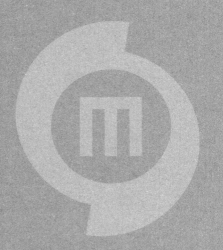

## CHAPTER 4

# The Formula for Fat Loss

"Meat for strength, vegetables for health." Wise words from Pavel Tsatsouline, the man responsible for bringing the Russian kettlebell craze to America, but I would add: "Meat plus vegetables for fat loss."

It's hard to overemphasize the importance of protein in the MetaShred Diet. It has both immediate and long-term impacts on hormones that regulate fat loss and your ability to build, maintain, and repair muscle (your number one calorie-burner).

The MetaShred Diet is serious about protein, and you'll need to be serious about getting it at every meal and snack. But, with all of the recipes that you'll have at your fingertips, I've made it as easy as possible for you.

Of course, there's more to the MetaShred Diet than just eating protein. In fact, every component of it is based on the latest rapid fat-loss science. In this chapter, I'll take you through every detail and show you why it's not only safe but also incredibly effective.

## Protein: Don't Believe the Haters

Before we get into all the good about protein, you might have some apprehensions about eating lots of this nutrient. There are some pretty nasty protein rumors floating around that claim high amounts of protein can negatively impact your health. So I'm going to set the record straight and give you the truth about four of the most pervasive protein myths.

# Myth 1. You're Eating Too Much Protein Already

One of the most common antiprotein cries you will hear is that people are already getting too much protein. You'll then be told that women only need 46 grams of protein each day and men only need 56 grams.

This is true. If you're only interested in getting enough protein so that you don't become ill from protein malnutrition, then please limit your protein intake to no more than 46 or 56 grams, respectively, per day. That amount of protein is *necessary*. However, if you're looking to get ripped without constantly feeling like you're so hungry that you could eat shoe leather, you'll want to take a different approach. The MetaShred Diet isn't about preventing deficiency, it's about optimizing and maximizing your progress. And you need more protein to do that.

To understand the crux of this too-much-protein argument, it's important to understand how much the antiprotein crowd misunderstands the data they are spouting. The misunderstanding centers on the Recommended Dietary Allowances—or RDAs—and what they represent.

According to the Health and Medicine Division of the National Academies of Sciences, Engineering, and Medicine and the Food and Nutrition Board, an RDA is the average daily dietary intake level sufficient to meet the nutrient requirements of nearly all (97 to 98 percent) healthy individuals in a group.[1]

So what does that mean? In the case of protein, it's simply the amount that will deliver enough essential amino acids—the building blocks of protein that your body can't make itself—to keep most people from suffering from protein malnutrition. It's not the *optimal* amount, it's the *necessary* amount.

When the RDA for protein was determined, no consideration was taken as to the beneficial effects of protein on weight loss, blood pressure, satiety, or risk of diabetes. This is because the concept of the RDA was first developed during World War II, when the

United States was concerned with food rationing, so officials had to figure out the smallest amount of food people needed stateside—while still preventing malnutrition—so that they could send the rest of the food overseas to support the troops.

The food and nutrition landscape has changed a lot since 1943, when the first RDAs were accepted. And now people are looking to use protein to optimize their fitness and health. The RDA for protein is 100 percent useless in this area. Instead of leaning on the RDA, we are empowered by the lesser-known "acceptable macronutrient distribution ranges," or AMDRs. AMDRs are a piece of dietary guidance set by the Health and Medicine Division of the National Academies of Sciences, Engineering, and Medicine and the Food and Nutrition Board.

The AMDRs provide a range of intakes for protein, carbohydrates, and fats that can be used in healthful diets. The AMDR for protein is 10 to 35 percent. This means that if your protein intake makes up 10 to 35 percent of the total calories in your diet, it is considered healthful, and there are no known adverse health effects. This alphabet soup of acronyms can make your head start to spin, so I want you to know that you don't need to worry about calculating anything for the MetaShred Diet. I've done all of that work for you, and the protein intake is right where it needs to be for optimizing health and maximizing your fat loss.[2]

## Myth 2. Excessive Protein Is Bad for Your Kidneys

When you hear about the dangers of eating more protein, the health of your kidneys is often brought up. One of the major jobs of your kidneys is to handle the elimination of the by-products of protein metabolism. If you are eating more protein, you will have more by-products, and thus your kidneys will need to work harder to filter and excrete more compounds. This is why people with kidney disease need to be careful with their protein intake.

In people with healthy kidneys, research shows that they can handle increased protein intake with no problem. In a 6-month-long clinical trial, scientists from the Department of

Human Nutrition at the University of Copenhagen in Denmark compared the impact of high-protein intakes (MetaShred Diet level) versus low-protein intakes (slightly below normal) on kidney function. They concluded that "moderate changes in dietary protein intake cause adaptive alterations in renal [kidney] cell size and function without the indication of adverse effects."[3]

This tells us that when you increase your protein intake, your kidneys adapt to their increased workload by growing and becoming more efficient. When you go the gym and lift more weights, your muscles adapt and grow. Adaptation and growth of your kidneys is a normal response by the human body—and not the fast track to being put on dialysis.

When looking at scientific research, the population being studied is very important. The impact of protein—at any level—in the diets of people with kidney disease is very different than people with normally functioning kidneys.

## Myth 3. Too Much Protein Is Bad for Your Liver

While your kidneys are responsible for excreting the by-products of protein metabolism, the actual metabolism of protein occurs in your liver. As with your kidneys, the idea that protein consumption is harmful to your liver is another case of applying findings from a sick population to those of a healthy population. People with liver disease have trouble metabolizing protein because their livers are damaged. But a healthy liver can metabolize as much protein as you can eat (within reason, of course). As Michael R. Charlton, MD, put it in the opening line of his article "Protein Metabolism and Liver Disease": "In health, the liver orchestrates the metabolism of proteins and amino acids. When the liver is diseased, the regulation of protein metabolism is frequently disturbed."[4]

## Myth 4. Eating More Protein Can Degrade Your Bones

The idea that protein can negatively impact bone health is a classic example of when a little knowledge of biochemistry is applied incorrectly on a large scale. When people eat more protein, it's common for researchers to observe an increase in calcium loss in study participants' urine. This is because your body breaks down protein into amino acids, and these amino acids can cause a decrease in the pH of your body. Your body responds to this by releasing minerals from your bones—for example, calcium—to bring the pH back up to where your body likes it. (Just as with blood sugar, your body likes to keep pH within a certain range.)

When you read the paragraph above, you may think, *Wow! Protein creates an acidic environment in my system, which causes my body to break down precious bone. Is this going to give me osteoporosis?*

No. This is part of the natural give-and-take that is constantly happening inside your body with every passing second. In fact, adding protein to your diet has been shown to be anabolic to your bones, meaning that it strengthens and builds them. There have been a handful of studies showing increased protein in the diet is associated with greater, not lower, mineral content in bones. In older people, higher protein intakes are also associated with lower risk of fractures.

In the review "Protein Intake and Bone Health," Jean-Philippe Bonjour, MD, succinctly puts an end to concerns about negative effects of protein on bone health, drawing this conclusion: "There is no evidence that high protein intake, per se, would be detrimental for bone mass and strength. Nevertheless, it appears reasonable to avoid very high protein diets when associated with low calcium intake."[5]

It isn't until your protein intake is three to four times what it should be—and your calcium intake is half of what it needs to be—that this might become an issue.

## Protein: Believe the Hype

Now that we've successfully debunked some of the biggest and baddest protein myths, let's shift our focus to how more protein is going to help you get better results as part of the MetaShred Diet.

As mentioned earlier, a major distinguishing factor between the calories in < calories out approach and the Carbohydrate-Insulin Hypothesis for weight loss is how the macronutrients—protein, carbohydrates, and fats—act in our bodies. In the former hypothesis, they are just sources of calories. But in the latter hypothesis, they are seen more as master hormonal switches. You'll see in this section that changing the amount of protein in your diet significantly changes the fat-loss environment in your body.

## Protein Helps You Feel Full

One of the great in-the-moment effects of protein is that it helps reduce hunger and increase fullness after a meal. It does this like a skilled puppeteer, pulling metabolic and hormonal strings throughout the digestive process to make you feel fuller longer, compared to if you had eaten carbohydrates or fat instead. Here are three of the strings it pulls.

## 1. Increased CCK

When protein leaves your stomach and hits the first part of your small intestine, this triggers the release of cholecystokinin, or CCK. CCK is a hormone that slows down the release of food from your stomach, while also traveling up to your brain, where it helps flip neuronal switches that tell you to stop eating. CCK is released in proportion to how much protein you consume: More protein means more CCK. CCK levels generally increase 15 minutes into a meal.

## 2. Increased PYY

Peptide YY, or PYY, is another hormone released by your small intestine when protein is ingested. It travels to the hypothalamic arcuate nucleus, a unique part of your brain that isn't fully behind the blood-brain barrier. It's like a little sentry outpost in your brain that has access to your bloodstream, where it can sense both hormones and nutrients in your circulation. PYY levels begin to rise 15 minutes into a meal and peak around 1.5 hours later.

PYY and PYY clones are being tested as antiobesity drugs. One study found that PYY injections led to a 30 percent reduction in calorie intake, while another study—which used a PYY nasal spray—only yielded minimal weight loss. I say let's skip the needles and nasal sprays and just opt for a protein-packed steak.

## 3. Decreased Ghrelin

CCK and PYY are part of the appetite alphabet soup that works to reduce appetite. But when it comes to increasing appetite, there's only one player in town: a hormone called ghrelin. And more ghrelin equals more hunger. Ghrelin is released from your stomach, and like CCK and PYY, it travels to your brain. But instead of getting you to stop eating, it coaxes your brain into telling you that you should eat more. The good news: Protein is very effective at decreasing ghrelin levels. So more protein equals less ghrelin and, ultimately, less hunger.

How much protein is needed to pull these metabolic strings? A common misconception about protein's ability to curb feelings of hunger is that any amount of protein will have this effect. This isn't the case. Not even close. Research from protein and satiety scientist Heather J. Leidy, PhD, shows that you need to eat 25 to 30 grams of protein to reap the benefits of protein for appetite reduction.[6]

If you eat protein beyond that amount, you will experience further increases in satiety, but you need to get over that initial hump of 25 to 30 grams for the satiation effect to kick in. I blame food marketing for driving this misconception about protein and increased fullness, as every product that contains 5 grams of protein is now being marketed as being "high" protein for curbing hunger. This just isn't the case. I've optimized the MetaShred Diet meals so that you can take advantage of the satiating effect of protein at each meal.

Before we move on to how to dial in the right amount of total daily protein for achieving a lean, muscular look, I want to share with you one rather remarkable study that sums up the powerful hunger-squashing effects of protein. David S. Weigle, MD, and other researchers at the University of Washington School of Medicine and the Oregon Health and Science University put 19 people on a traditional/normal protein diet geared toward maintaining the participants' weight for a 2-week period.[7] After this normal protein phase, the researchers kept the total calories of the diet the same, but shifted protein up and fat down so that protein was at the MetaShred Diet levels. Again, they were put on this new diet for 2 weeks, with calories controlled so that the subjects' body weights didn't fluctuate. To that point, this was a pretty standard nutrition study, but what happened next is where it got interesting.

In the third and final diet phase, the study participants remained on the higher-protein diet, but were given 15 percent more calories to eat each day. They were told to eat whenever they were hungry and to stop eating when they were satisfied. Basically, they could eat as much or as little of the diet that was given to them. Almost immediately, the average calorie intake of the study participants dropped by 440 calories per day. From then until the end of the study, 12 weeks later, the average weight loss was 8 pounds of fat.

Throughout different checkpoints during the study, the participants' metabolic rates—along with a collection of biomarkers in their blood—were measured. When the data was analyzed, it turned out that the subjects' metabolic rates stayed relatively stable. So the increased weight loss could not be attributed to protein increasing their daily calorie burn.

What changed was their leptin sensitivity. Leptin is a hormone that is released from fat cells and acts on the brain to reduce food intake. In this study, increasing protein intake made the participants' central nervous systems more sensitive to leptin. This allowed the same amount of leptin in their blood to have a greater ability to drive fullness and satiety.

I think this study is remarkable because:

1. It highlights the point that protein, carbohydrates, and fats are not just sources of calories, but that each of them impacts hormones and our bodies in unique ways.

**2.** Protein is such a powerful appetite suppressant that even when people were told to eat as much as they wanted, the high protein content of their diets had them opt for less food.

## Protein Helps Give You the "Look" after Weight Loss

When we examined traditional rapid weight-loss solutions in Chapter 23, it was clear that most of the approaches didn't work. Those that did focused purely on indiscriminately and massively cutting calories. (Remember very low calorie diets?)

The best way to describe how you look after one of these protocols is "skinny-fat." The skinny-fat look is the result of losing large amounts of fat *and* muscle while you're dieting. You are smaller and skinnier but lack the definition and *look* that you were hoping for. That's because this look is driven by having an appreciable amount of muscle on your body. When you diet down, your body goes into conservation mode and—without the adequate biological signal—it will break down and burn your muscle for energy.

Protein helps provide this needed signal to your body. Specifically, I'm talking about what scientists call muscle protein synthesis (MPS). Like the name sounds, this is the synthesis—or building—of the proteins that make up your muscles. Bodybuilders and weight lifters have intuitively known for decades that eating more protein leads to bigger and stronger muscles. But how that happens—and how to optimize that process—was unknown for a long time.

Thanks to protein researchers like Donald K. Layman, PhD, an emeritus professor of nutrition at the University of Illinois, and Doug Paddon-Jones, PhD, at the University of Texas Medical Branch, we now know that there's a specific building block found in all protein—and especially abundant in animal proteins—that flips the cellular switch that activates MPS. This building block is an amino acid called leucine. When you eat protein, leucine ignites the process of MPS, and your body then uses it and the other amino acids as the raw materials from which to build proteins into muscle.

The more often we can turn on MPS, the greater our ability to build, repair, and maintain our muscle mass while dieting. When we look at the "+3 squares a day" framework of the MetaShred Diet (see opposite page), we will look more closely at Dr. Paddon-Jones's work, which elucidates how amount and timing of your protein consumption can optimize this effect.

## Protein Helps Curb Your Sweet Tooth with Jedi Mind Tricks

Wouldn't it be nice if all you needed to do was look in the mirror, wave your hand in front of yourself, à la Obi-Wan Kenobi, and say: "This isn't the Chicago-style pizza you are craving . . . " And wham! You can stand in front of that decadent pepperoni-filled deep-dish pizza with no desire to look at it, let alone eat it.

That would be nice, but it isn't happening anytime soon. In lieu of actual Jedi mind tricks, protein is your best bet. How? According to a 2011 study that employed functional brain scans, having a protein-rich meal can make your brain less interested in reward-driven foods like pizza, french fries, cakes, cookies, and pies.[8]

While the exact mechanism in which protein goes about having this effect is unknown, it appears that eating 24 to 50 grams of protein—think eggs, dairy, beef, pork, chicken, and fish—has sustained effects on food cravings for as long as 3 hours after eating a meal. When exposed to pictures of decadent foods that everyone craves, the researchers discovered that there is reduced activation in the areas of your brain associated with both food cravings (insula) and rewards (prefrontal).

This is as close to a Jedi mind trick as we're going to get and yet another powerful reason that the MetaShred Diet is powered by protein.

## Protein Enhances Fat Loss

When you take into account all of the above factors, it's easy to see that eating MetaShred Diet levels of protein will increase fat loss and help you maintain your muscle mass while dieting. When pitted up against normal protein diets, higher-protein diets are consistently the superior tool for fat loss. Now, let's look at how to optimize the timing and amount of protein in your diet with the MetaShred Diet "+3 squares a day" approach to meal planning.

## Your New Eating Schedule

The MetaShred Diet uses what I call "+3 squares a day" meal frequency. There are lots of theories on the origins of a "square meal." Perhaps it comes from the square wooden plates that sailors used. Or maybe it denotes meals that contained four food groups, with each group representing the side of a square. Regardless of where it came from, a square meal is thought to be a complete, nutritious meal.

Of course, a classic recommendation is to eat three square meals a day for good health. But as mentioned previously, for the last couple of decades, the fitness community has been touting six to eight meals a day to boost your metabolism. (Don't forget: That's total bunk.) Even though six to eight meals is what many people still advise, other experts recommend three meals, four meals, or two meals; or to eat your meals only during certain windows of time during the day; or even to eat zero meals, as part of an intermittent fasting regimen.

How can you make sense of this, and what should you do?

This is where +3 squares a day comes into play. It's the answer you've been looking for—simple, effective, and easy to implement. It takes into account a wide scope of research that includes time-based feeding and satiety studies, and the biology of muscle protein synthesis.

The premise is this: You eat breakfast, lunch, and dinner every day. This is the "3 squares" part. In addition, you have a protein-rich snack, and, on days that you exercise intensely, you have a protein shake mixed in water. This is the "+" part. Now, let me tell you why it works so well.

# The Ugly Truth about Eating More Often

In a 2003 interview with *Rolling Stone* magazine, Steve Jobs stressed the importance of recognizing the unintended consequences of our actions, saying, "There are downsides to everything; there are unintended consequences to everything. The most corrosive piece of technology that I've ever seen is called television—but then again, television, at its best, is magnificent."[9]

With nutrition, we often overlook the unintended consequences of changes that we make with our diets. Protein is often touted as the greatest part of any diet, but eating more and more protein eventually leads to the displacement of other foods that contain unique and essential nutrients, such as fruits, vegetables, and fibrous grains.

When it comes to meal frequency, all of the focus was on the straw man of metabolism enhancement, without any thought to what happens when you're actually eating these smaller, more-frequent meals. So let's do that now.

Since eating more often doesn't impact your metabolism, what exactly are the benefits? The one that's most often cited is greater satiety and fullness. The line of thinking here is that when you eat smaller meals more often, you're going to be more satiated and feel less hungry during the day. Also, by eating small meals more often, you'll stabilize your blood glucose levels, preventing the dips in blood sugar that increase your drive to eat.

This brings us to more work by Dr. Leidy, who put this meal frequency/satiety broscience to the test to see if eating more actually does make you less hungry during the day. She took study participants and allowed them either three meals per day or six meals per day. The total amount of calories for the day was the same for each group, regardless of how many meals they were eating.[10]

The six-meals-per-day approach failed miserably. The problem was that when they chopped 2,100 calories up into six meals, the meals were too small to be satisfying. For someone who is dieting, this problem only gets worse. That's because as you lose fat and get closer to your goal, you need to eat fewer and fewer calories in order to continue your progress. As a result, your small meals will then become smaller and smaller.

So when people crank up the number of meals they are eating in the name of boosting their metabolisms, the unintended consequence is that they are making their meals so small, they're never full. From a satiety standpoint, fewer but larger meals are the way to go.

## Time-Based Protein Power

You can make protein even more powerful by consuming it at the right times. But, to understand how to optimize your protein intake during the day, it's important to first understand how the average person eats this nutrient throughout the day.

When you look at protein from a meal-based perspective, you'll see that people generally have what researchers call a skewed protein distribution during the day. They eat a small amount of protein at breakfast, slightly more—but still very little—at lunch, and then a massive amount of protein at dinner. Dr. Paddon-Jones—one of the top protein researchers mentioned earlier—observed this and wanted to see if this was the best way to maximize muscle protein synthesis. He wanted to know if you eat more protein at a meal, do you get increased MPS?

So he put together a test to answer the question. In the study, people ate either a ground beef patty containing 30 grams of protein or several ground beef patties containing a total of 90 grams of protein.[11] What he found surprised a lot of people: Muscle protein synthesis was increased the same in both groups. Whether people ate 30 grams or 90 grams of protein, they experienced about a 46 percent increase in muscle protein synthesis. The upshot: There seemed to be a ceiling to how much protein was needed to maximize MPS at a given meal.

The next big follow-up question Dr. Paddon-Jones and his colleagues had was this: What would happen if you took the same amount of protein that people eat in their traditional skewed distribution, but spread it out evenly across the day to ensure that they consume 30 grams of protein at each meal? The idea was to see if this strategy increased MPS, even though the participants would be eating the same total amount of protein as usual.

The results: The researchers found that an even distribution of protein—where people ate 30 grams of protein at all meals—yielded a 25 percent increase in MPS across the entire day, compared to when participants ate in their normal fashion.[12] So, yes, the total amount of protein you eat matters, but it also matters how you eat your protein throughout the day.

## The Peaks and Valleys of Eating Protein

If eating 30 grams of protein at every meal boosts the muscle-building effect of protein, would eating more meals result in even better results? The answer is no.

As researchers further delved into the question about the optimal amount of protein needed to maximize muscle building and repair, they found that in order for our muscles to properly and accurately sense the amino acids and protein, they needed to come in peaks and valleys.[13] That is, protein levels in your blood need to peak and then decrease back down to a valley.

You can't just have nonstop protein barraging your muscles. They essentially become desensitized to it. Think about when you get a cut. It hurts when it happens, but then the pain subsides. You are still cut, but your body has desensitized itself to the pain signal. So you no longer feel the same discomfort that you did when you were initially cut.

When it comes to your muscles and protein, 4 hours is the closest you want to eat two protein-rich meals while still being able to maximize this effect. One caveat: protein shakes. Liquid protein is digested faster than protein from solid food. So the amino acids from, say, a whey protein shake peak and then subside in your bloodstream more quickly. Because of this, you can have a protein shake 2 hours after a meal and still get the optimal effect.[14]

The timing of protein and its ability to maximize the signals needed to build and repair your muscles are another reason why the +3 squares a day works so well. It spreads your meals far enough apart throughout the day so that you can give your body the protein peaks and valleys that it needs. I've also optimized the protein content of the meals in the MetaShred Diet to ensure that you will have the balanced distribution that Dr. Paddon-Jones and his colleagues found works so well.

## The Genius Way to Snack

A protein-rich snack is a key part of the MetaShred Diet. It helps control your food cravings and manage your hunger throughout the day. You have the freedom to put that snack anywhere you would like during the day, depending on your schedule and hunger levels. The two most common times that my clients choose to eat their snacks is between lunch and dinner or after dinner. Use the guide that follows to determine which time is right for you.

## When to Choose a Midafternoon Snack

This is a good time to snack, as it's when people generally have an energy lull during the day. A snack at this time can pep up your willpower and motivation to help you power through the rest of your day. Having a midafternoon snack also prevents you from being over-hungry at dinner. This is especially true if you eat an early lunch and then a late dinner. By the time you sit down to eat your last meal of the day, your enhanced level of hunger—combined with the accumulation of stress from the day—might leave you eating more than you were planning. The midafternoon snack can help take the edge off and save you from compulsively overeating at dinner.

## When to Choose an Evening Snack

Having your snack after dinner is good for people who are late-night snackers. Over the years, I've found that the time when people consume the highest number of unaccounted calories is after dinner and before bed. If this sounds like you, then placing your MetaShred snack post-dinner will allow you to still snack at night, but in a way that won't negatively impact your fat-loss results.

## Does It Matter What Time of Day You Eat?

Aside from spreading out your main meals at least 4 hours apart, it doesn't matter when you eat them. You don't have to eat breakfast immediately upon rising, but I recommend that you eat it within 1 to 2 hours of waking. Likewise, there isn't a magic cutoff point at night when you need to stop eating. So if you don't get home until 9:00 p.m., and then you don't eat dinner until 10:00, that's fine. There's no need to find a new job so that you can eat dinner at 7:00 p.m. Your body digests food very well while you are sleeping, and research shows that you can build and repair muscle during your evening slumber. The timing of your meals, outside of your postworkout protein shake—I'll explain this more in the meal plans—should be more geared toward convenience and whatever will allow you to execute your plan most consistently.

In Chapter 6, I'll give you all the details you need for selecting the meals for your plan and what foods are in them.

## The Truth about Carbohydrates

A big problem with nutrition is that the advice is often very extreme. There rarely seems to be a middle ground. For example, many experts recommend a high-carb, low-fat diet, while others claim that a low-carb, high-fat diet is the only answer. Where is the in-between?

The MetaShred Diet is that in-between. That's because:

1. It contains the right amount and type of carbohydrate to fuel your body's energy needs.

2. It provides you with an adequate volume of food so that you're satisfied after a meal.

3. It limits your total carbohydrates in order to create a hormonal environment that speeds fat loss.

Before I can really talk about low-carb versus low-fat diets, and how we need to create a hybrid of them for optimal fat loss, I have to set the record straight. I hear all the time that low-carb diets are bad for you—from physicians, dieticians, personal trainers, and even the guy at the UPS store. The truth is, there is no clinical data to show that removing a small or even a significant amount of carbohydrates from your diet is unhealthy. Low-carbohydrate diets are not bad for your health. It's quite the opposite: They're actually good for you. That's a position that's based on what we know from actual research and not misinformed Internet articles, Facebook debaters, or decades-old dogma.

## Low Carb versus Low Fat

The funny thing about the low-carb versus low-fat argument is that both diets work if you execute them properly. You can absolutely lose weight on a low-fat diet; people have been doing it for decades. And there is scientific data to show that low-fat diets do work.

But do they work better than low-carb diets? Probably not. Part of this is the fact that executing a low-fat diet is hard for people to do over the long-term. Fat makes food taste good, and it makes you feel more full after a meal. Being tasty and filling are two key components to a diet that lasts. I'm pretty sure no one has ever asked for "the bland diet with meals that leave you hungry after you eat them."

When you add to this the hard truth that we don't move around as much as we used to and that we're much more sedentary with every passing day, lower-carbohydrate diets begin to look like a more appealing option. The less active we are, the less proficient our bodies are going to be at using carbohydrates.

When you look at research that pits low-carb diets against low-fat diets, after 6 months low-carb diets will generally lead to 9 pounds greater weight loss. Unfortunately, at 12 months low-carb and low-fat diets are shown to be equally effective. That is to say, neither is particularly effective. My interpretation of what happens between 6 and 12 months has less to do with biology and more to do with human behavior.[15]

In clinical trials, the support given to study participants becomes significantly less at the 6-month mark, leaving people to their own devices. This manifests itself in the form of reduced compliance. The less compliant you are to a diet, the less likely you are to reap the benefits of that diet. And thus, the results from low-carb and low-fat diets begin to look more and more the same. What's more, the actual compositions of the diets that are being eaten by the study participants begin to look more and more similar.

Execution is key, and the more extreme you get with your diet—whether it's lower fat or lower carb—the harder it becomes to execute on a consistent basis. With the MetaShred Diet, I've restricted the carbohydrates enough to give you the hormonal benefits, but not so much that it limits food options and becomes harder for you to eat this way.

## The Hierarchy of Carbohydrates

This is the guiding principle for carbohydrates in the MetaShred Diet. It will also be a valuable tool for you as you transition off the MetaShred Diet and head out into the nutritional wild.

The hierarchy of carbohydrates is a concept that I came up with in response to the recurring questions of, "Should I stop eating [insert any carbohydrate-containing food]?" Fundamentally, it's nearly impossible to single out one food in your diet as being *bad* such that you should stop eating it. Most things in your diet are relative, so singling out mangoes as *the* carbohydrate that you should remove from your diet is impossible, unless we know what other carbs you are eating. This is where the hierarchy of carbohydrates comes in to be your decision-making savior.

**Foods with added sugars**
**Refined grains**
**Whole grains/starches**
**Fruit**
**Vegetables**
**Green vegetables**

With the hierarchy of carbohydrates, the foods are listed in descending order of carbohydrate density. So a refined grain-based food is going to have more carbohydrates per serving than a serving of green vegetables. This also means that they're listed in ascending order of volume. You can eat a larger amount of green vegetables for a given amount of carbohydrates than if you were to eat that same amount of whole grain-based carbohydrates. As an added side benefit, the foods on the lower end of the hierarchy of carbohydrates generally contain more nutrients than the foods on the upper end of the hierarchy.

When eating for fat loss, you want to eat more food from the bottom of the list and less food from the top. If you wanted to reduce the amount of carbohydrates in your diet, you start from the top down, as that will give you the biggest bang, while allowing you to eat the largest volume of food. Remember, the volume of food that you eat is a big determinant of how satisfied you are after a meal.

I've already built this into the MetaShred Diet recipes, meals plans, and diet phase shifts, but having this guide in your nutritional tool belt will be very valuable in life after the scripted diet phases of the MetaShred Diet end.

## Secret Sauce: The Diet-Exercise Connection

I know this is a diet book, but I would be doing you a disservice if I didn't discuss exercise. Exercise is such an integral part of not just rapid fat loss, but also getting the end result that you want. As I wrote earlier, maintaining your muscle while dieting is one of the biggest factors in determining how you look after you lose 10, 20, 30, or more pounds.

While many of my clients have a goal in mind when it comes to their ideal scale weight, their more powerful benchmark for success is a specific look that they want to achieve. Everyone can have a different look in mind, but the foundation of this look is always that a person's muscles are covered with minimal fat. No client has ever asked to lose weight in hopes that they look like one of the 36 men at the end of Ancel Keys's landmark 1940s Minnesota Starvation Experiment.[16]

When you diet, your body becomes thrifty, always looking for ways to cut expenditures. In the case of your body, its expenditures are not financial, but caloric. One of the biggest expenses in your body's metabolic balance sheet is muscle. Muscle, unlike fat, requires significant caloric expense for upkeep and usage. This is one of the reasons that having a fair amount of muscle can make dieting easier: It gives you the ability to easily burn more calories.

When dieting, your body will gladly burn up some of the proteins that make up a muscle—if it deems it necessary. And this is most likely to be muscle that gets the least use. But one of the main benefits of exercise when you're dieting—and this is especially true in regard to resistance training—is that it lets your body know that all of the muscle that you currently have is essential. So it can't afford to get rid of any in the name of reducing your daily calorie needs. You might say that exercise protects your muscle and forces your body to use more excess body fat for energy.

## Increase Demands to Increase Results

You already know that your body builds muscle in response to lifting weights. The mechanism is simple: After each training session—during the recovery process—your body works to become stronger so that it can better handle your next workout. It's called adaptation, and it's survival of the fittest 101.

And when you're dieting, this same mechanism is what keeps your body from breaking down muscle for calories. You get your body to hold on to your muscle by *using* your muscle.

The best way to test this concept would be if we could create such a restricted caloric environment that muscle loss would be a forgone conclusion. Then, we would be able to focus on the ability of exercise to prevent the loss of muscle. Fortunately, a group of researchers at West Virginia University ran this exact study.[17]

There were 20 people enrolled in the study. Half of the participants were placed in an aerobic exercise group. They completed four exercise sessions per week, working their way up to 50 to 60 minutes of the aerobic exercise of their choice at each session. The other half of the study participants were placed in a circuit-training group. This group completed only three exercise sessions per week. Each session was a total body-weight training routine done in a circuit. Both groups were placed on an extremely miserable 800-calorie-per-day liquid diet for the duration of the 12-week study.

At the end of the study, the group that did circuit-training lost more weight than the aerobic exercise group—32 pounds of total fat—maintained all of their muscle mass, and also maintained their metabolic rates. The aerobic exercise group lost 9 pounds of muscle, which resulted in an average reduction of metabolic rate equal to 211 calories per day.

# THE WORKOUTS THAT SPEED YOUR RESULTS

You can approach your exercise training in many ways. I recommend a mix of weight training and interval cardio training. You could accomplish this with three workouts a week of total bodyweight training and two separate workouts of intervals. This is a classic approach that will allow you to focus on strength and muscle on your lifting days, and serious cardio training on your interval days. In fact, if you go into the gym and work your whole body hard with weights for 45 minutes to an hour, you'll get the benefits you want. Add the cardio on your "off" days, and you're set.

But you might prefer to bundle both of these methods into a single workout. Maybe you're also time-crunched. My colleague BJ Gaddour, the fitness director at *Men's Health* and creator of the MetaShred fitness program, now has two great options.

The first is the 21-DAY METASHRED. This provides nine 30-minute total-body workouts that you do 3 days a week. It's best for people who want to get the most out of limited time to train or haven't done much high-intensity exercise. (It'll change that in a hurry.) You can get this at www.21DayMetaShred.com.

The second option is METASHRED EXTREME. This gives you a total of eight 40-minute workouts that you do four times a week. (Plus, there are a ton of bonus routines that let you amp your fitness even more and also work out more frequently, if desired.) In this one, you'll train your upper body one day and then your lower body the next. That makes it even better for building muscle, while still giving you an incredible cardio challenge. You can learn more and order this program at www.metashredextreme.com.

The results you get when you combine the MetaShred Diet with one of the MetaShred fitness programs can be astounding.

This study shows that even when put in the most extreme dieting situation, rigorous circuit-training can put the brakes on muscle loss and ensure maintenance of a robust metabolic rate. By adding resistance training while on the MetaShred Diet, you can increase the demand on your muscles—forcing your body to hold on to those muscles, which will then accelerate your progress. (See "The Workouts That Speed Your Results" above.)

# Exercise as a Drug

Exercise is an incredible drug. For a short period of time, it essentially allows you to specify what your body does with the food you are putting into it. Sound too good to be true? It isn't.

When you exercise, your muscles become carbohydrate sponges. That's because your muscles have special sugar transporters that get stimulated when you work out. These transporters move to the surface of your muscle cells, ready to soak up any sugar they can find. This influx of sugar transporters on your muscle cells—which is driven by exercise—is muscle-specific. It doesn't happen with your fat cells.

This is the first nutritional advantage that you get with exercise, and some research suggests that it can last upward of 24 hours. But it's at its strongest directly following exercise.

One of the reasons that we want to send sugars to our muscles is because, once they get in there, they're trapped. Your muscles are rather "selfish," and they have no ability to release sugar back out to your body once it is inside them. So that muscle alone will use the sugar for energy. If your body needs more energy for other activities or processes, it has to rely on your liver—which stores a small amount of sugar—and your fat cells (which is exactly what you want!).

You'll also be happy to know that this isn't an all-or-nothing proposition. It doesn't only happen when you go to the gym and go all out for an hour. The simple act of going for a walk after dinner can increase this effect as well.

It's truly powerful stuff. Despite the best efforts of scientists and pharmaceutical companies, there are no drugs available that can selectively shuttle carbohydrates to muscle like exercise can. And the only co-pay required is your effort.

I realize that sometimes the energy dips that can happen on a diet can make the couch or elevator look especially attractive. But fight the urge, and stay as active as you can. One extra workout can have a positive impact on your body's ability to process and use the carbs that you're eating.

## Boost Your Muscle-Building Signals

As mentioned earlier, protein has the special ability to turn on muscle building at the molecular level. Exercise has that same effect. And if you combine exercise and protein, you get even stronger and more sustained muscle-building signals.

Just as protein helps you lose weight via a variety of pathways, exercise helps you maximize the use of the protein that you're eating. Arguably, the older you are, the more effective exercise is at facilitating the relationship between the protein you eat and your muscles.

Exercise helps your muscles better sense the presence of amino acids, allowing for above-average levels of muscle protein synthesis without more protein. Exercise does this by the following ways:

1. **It improves blood vessel function.** This allows your blood vessels to stretch and expand so that more nutrient-rich blood can travel to your muscles. As a side benefit, blood vessel function is an exciting area of cardiovascular disease research. Improving blood vessel function seems to reduce your risk of heart disease.

2. **It improves nutrient delivery.** Exercise also helps "open" your muscles at a cellular level so that more blood can actually get into your muscles. The result is a faster and more efficient delivery of amino acids into your muscles.

3. **It improves muscle-building signals.** The muscle-building signals that are activated by protein in your muscles are like light switches. They are either on or off. Once a light switch is on, you can't turn it on more. But you can ensure that it stays on longer. This is what exercise does. It allows the protein that you eat to turn the muscle-building signals on in your body for longer periods of time.

The beauty of the relationship between protein and exercise, and the benefits outlined above, is that this isn't just an immediate nutritional fling. It is a longer-term relationship with sustained effects, upward of 24 hours.

In the MetaShred Diet, you consume a simple protein shake shortly after exercise so that you can start taking advantage of this process immediately. This is to also give you another opportunity during the day—outside of your meals and snacks—to boost muscle protein synthesis. But know that the benefits of exercise and how your body uses protein are sustained. So you don't need to go into a cold sweat if you can't slam a whey protein shake the second you're finished lifting weights. The benefit will still be there, even if you're delayed for a bit.

This is a useful way to look at all aspects of this diet. Follow it as best you can, but realize that an effective diet is really about consistency. If you have trouble getting the right amount of protein at a meal, or you eat too many calories at another, don't stress out about it. Just move on and look for ways to plan better and stay on course in the future. In the next chapter, I'll show you how to do just that.

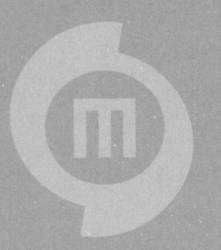

## CHAPTER 5

# The Lifestyle X-Factors

Your sleep quality, stress levels, and social circles are all lifestyle factors that can significantly impact your weight-loss results. They're also often ignored on most weight-loss programs. While eating the right number of calories is imperative to your success, all of these variables can seriously affect your ability to do that. What's more, when you focus on optimizing these areas, you can literally speed fat loss even more. I'll show you how.

## Sleep: The Real Secret to Fat Loss?

It's very common for people to have a little trouble sleeping when they embark on an aggressive fat-loss program. That's because some of the hormonal effects of fat-loss activities run counter to the hormonal environment needed for optimal sleep. Cutting calories and attacking your exercise sessions can lead to an increase in catecholamines. Catecholamines are your "fight-or-flight" hormones. These compounds were historically used to heighten awareness and reaction time and increase muscular activity so that you could fight or run away from a dangerous situation.

Hundreds of years ago, catecholamines were great for survival, but for the modern man or woman, they are great for fat loss. They help drive the breakdown and release of stored body fat from your fat cells into your bloodstream where it can be used for energy.

Both rigorous exercise and the additional stress and food vigilance associated with an intense diet can cause increases in catecholamine levels. Unfortunately, as you can imagine, hormones that increase awareness, reaction time, and muscular activity don't help with sleep. This is why sleep can be an issue with rapid fat-loss achievers.

Without the added hormonal challenges that rapid fat loss brings to getting sleep, people are already pretty poor sleepers. According to the Centers for Disease Control and Prevention, one-third of Americans get less than 7 hours of sleep on a daily basis. Contrast this to a 1998 survey that found that one-third of Americans were getting 8 hours of sleep or less each night. We're getting less and less sleep.[1]

Another survey by the National Sleep Foundation found that 40 percent of men and 49 percent of women have trouble falling asleep at least once a week.[2] As a society, we often wear minimal sleep as a badge of honor, pushing us to work longer and longer hours, which leads to less and less sleep. Arianna Huffington, a champion for the benefits of sleep, didn't see the importance of sleep until she was so sleep-deprived that she passed out while working—and hit her head on her desk so hard that she broke her cheekbone.

Consistently getting 8 to 9 hours of sleep each night could be one of the best things you can do for your waistline. Lack of sleep increases your drive to eat more and move less on multiple levels. Many researchers believe that there is a relationship between decreased sleep time—less than 8 hours per night—and increased body weight.[3] This relationship is clear in children and adolescents, but less clear in adults, mainly because there's not enough high-quality data to make the conclusion.

However, the mechanisms and behaviors that link lack of sleep to weight gain are pretty obvious. Just look at how sleep impacts many factors that contribute to obesity.

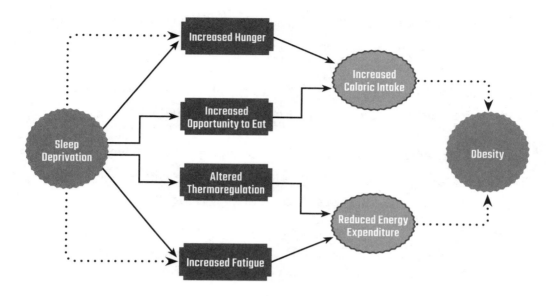

## Snooze Less, Eat More

There's no question that sleeping less sets up your biology so that you will be driven to eat more. It does so with respect to hormonal changes that increase hunger and behavioral changes that give you more opportunities to eat. Those aren't the beginnings of a recipe for fat-loss success.

One piece of traditional, long-standing, weight-loss advice is to not eat after 8:00 p.m. (or 7:00 or 9:00, depending on who you ask). The genesis of this advice is flawed, as it was based on the idea that your body doesn't digest and metabolize food while you sleep. This is totally untrue. However, for many, eating at night is an unregulated source of calories. So curtailing this behavior can be the difference between losing and not losing fat. It's an example of advice that can work, but for the wrong reason.

In 2006, Professor Michael Sivak, PhD, from the University of Michigan, published a viewpoint piece in the journal *Obesity Reviews* entitled, "Sleeping More as a Way to Lose Weight."[4] In this article, Dr. Sivak proposed a simplified look at eating and sleeping, which calculated "calories per hour awake." This showed that by going to sleep 1 hour earlier, a person would reduce his caloric intake by 6 percent.

At its most basic level, this shows that the longer you're awake, the more chances you have to eat. I love the simplicity of Dr. Sivak's argument, and I find it to be enhanced by these three reasons, which show why night eating is particularly problematic.

1. **Poor food choices.** Research shows that at night, people generally snack on high-fat, high-carbohydrate foods.[5] These kinds of foods are easily accessed—no prep or cooking needed—and easy to consume. (Did I just eat that whole bag of tortilla chips?)

2. **Stress eating.** I have observed that eating after dinner is unregulated and generally an unrecognized source of calories in my clients. Eating is a form of stress relief for people, and eating at night is often used to help take the edge off the day's stress so that one can get to sleep.

3. **Mindless eating.** Eating while playing games on your phone or while watching TV leaves you less satisfied, less full, and more likely to eat more. At night, when you are looking to zone out a little, you can be more apt to snack in an unregulated fashion while doing those activities.

## How Sleep Affects Fat-Loss Hormones

How long and how well you sleep can have a major impact on hormones that regulate your appetite and ability to burn fat. The two hormones most readily impacted by a lack of sleep are leptin and ghrelin.

Ghrelin, your primary hunger hormone, is increased when you don't get enough shut-eye. This results in an enhanced drive to eat. How much ghrelin is increased and how much more you will eat were two research questions that Josiane Broussard, PhD, of the Sleep and Chronobiology Laboratory at the University of Colorado in Boulder, set out to answer. Dr. Broussard devised a clinical trial that took a group of young men who normally got 8 hours of sleep and exposed them to 4 nights of limited sleep—just 4.5 hours per night. After the fourth night, she gave them unlimited access to lunch and dinner buffets.[6]

The impact: Ghrelin levels were significantly increased when the study participants were sleep-restricted. And the number of calories from sweet snacks that participants ate at dinner was directly related to the increase in ghrelin levels—meaning that when these people were the hungriest, they were drawn to sugary snacks, not spinach.

The drive to eat more sugary foods when ghrelin levels are increased is right in line with the findings of a 2016 study published in *Neuropsychopharmacology*. The researchers found a link between ghrelin levels and impulsive behavior.[7]

Now, think about how this might apply to you: Imagine that you're on a diet plan and adhering to it well. But then you have a big deadline at work, so you stay up late a few nights, reducing your sleep. Even though you're putting forth your best effort to stick to your diet plan, ghrelin is working against you—increasing your hunger and making you more likely to impulsively binge on a box of cookies.

What's more, you may experience this effect after just a single night of burning the midnight oil. While Dr. Broussard's study consisted of 4 days of sleep restriction, a 2008 study in the *Journal of Sleep Research* reported that just 1 night of inadequate shut-eye resulted in a 22 percent increase in ghrelin levels.[8]

Leptin is another fat-loss hormone that's drastically impacted by shortened sleep. Leptin is a hormone released by your fat cells that helps curb appetite, enhance metabolic rate, and regulate how much stored fat you burn. So you want leptin working in your favor. And of all the factors that can impact this hormone, sleep is one of the most profound.

Researchers from the University of Chicago found that restricting 1 night of sleep to 4 hours can yield an 18 percent decrease in leptin levels—with a corresponding 24 percent increase in hunger and a 23 percent increase in appetite.[9] The negative changes in leptin levels due to insufficient sleep reach beyond hunger, as they may also be the driving force behind the reduction in insulin sensitivity—your body's ability to process and use carbohydrates—that also occurs with lack of sleep.[10]

## Why You Need to Sleep to Burn More Calories

I'm sure you don't need a 10-page research paper from the journal *Sleep* to tell you that sleeping less leads to fatigue and a cranky attitude. (But in case you were wondering, there is one.) Pretty much everyone knows that lack of sleep causes fatigue and performance deficiencies, but the worst part is that you stop being aware of these ill-effects after a couple of days. You actually get used to functioning in a fatigued state, yet you don't realize that you're overtired and not performing at your best. Sleep-deprived fatigue becomes your new normal.

One of the biggest downsides to this fatigue is that it will make you burn fewer calories. This is because you'll tend to move less during the day and also because your body will become more conservative with the number of calories you burn overall. Both of these occurrences are a huge barrier to rapid fat loss, as they are the total opposite of what you need to happen. You need greater energy output, and you need your body to become more frivolous, not conservative, with the amount of calories that it burns each day.

How does inadequate sleep cause you to burn fewer calories during the day? It causes changes to your metabolism, particularly your resting metabolic rate and postmeal calorie burning. Resting metabolic rate is essentially the total amount of calories that you burn each day if you were to lie in bed all day. When you don't get enough sleep, this amount is decreased—putting you behind the eight ball before the day even starts.

After you eat a meal, your body's metabolism ramps up. It burns more calories, especially if you have a higher-protein meal, as it digests and processes the foods that you eat. When you aren't getting enough sleep, this postmeal metabolic bump can be 20 percent lower.

As fatigue increases with sleep deprivation, you can imagine that your motivation to be more active will wane as well. Even if you honor your commitments and complete all of your workouts, you'll still move less during the day. Studies involving sleep deprivation and daily activity have shown that getting just 5.5 hours of sleep per night can lead to a 33 percent reduction in total activity for the day.[11, 12]

## Get a Great Night's Sleep

If you want to maximize your results on the MetaShred Diet, you need to get 7 to 9 hours of sleep each night. The MetaShred Diet is all about getting the various systems in your body to work together so that you can maximize fat burning. But with insufficient sleep, you'll guarantee that your body will be working against you.

I believe there are several strategies to getting great sleep, which I've compiled into a list for you. I hope that you implement them all, but if you choose to use only one, please pick number eight, as I think it provides the most benefit.

### 1. Have a Bedtime Routine

Much of falling asleep at night is psychological. Even the classic warm glass of milk, which people consistently report as an effective sleep aid, seems to be more of a psychological help than a physiological one. Many people have trouble falling asleep at night. Creating a nightly ritual signals your body that it's time to start winding down. This doesn't just mean doing the same things each night before you go to sleep, but also going to sleep and waking up around the same time, day in and day out. The consistency of simple sleep/wake times also has benefits with respect to your sleep biology, as it helps optimize your circadian rhythm.

### 2. Avoid Alcohol before Bed

Having a nightcap before you go to sleep may seem like a good idea, as alcohol is a physiological depressant that causes your body to relax. But alcohol is bad for sleep. You might then wonder, if alcohol is a relaxant, how could it be bad for sleep? Alcohol will help you get to sleep faster—what sleep researchers call decreasing sleep onset latency—but you're more likely to wake up in the middle of the night.

Alcohol also reduces the total percentage of your sleep that is REM sleep. REM, or rapid eye movement, sleep is the holy grail of shut-eye. During REM sleep, your brain works to enhance its memory, creativity, and sensory processing. My advice is don't drink for several hours before bed, to ensure that your body has the time needed to process and metabolize all of the alcohol in your system before it's time to hit the hay.

## 3. Avoid Stimulants

Just as you should avoid physiological depressants, like alcohol, before sleep, you should also be wary of any stimulants that you're consuming. Caffeine is the most commonly consumed drug in the world, and many people don't think to audit their caffeine consumption when they're having trouble sleeping. Start by limiting caffeine in any form— coffee, energy drinks, soda—starting at 4:00 p.m. And then move back from there—2:00, noon, and so on—until you can effectively fall asleep. (Somewhere between 2:00 and 4:00 p.m. seems to be the sweet spot for most people.)

## 4. Unplug

Power down your phone, turn off the TV, put away your laptop, and take a deep breath. The light emitted from TVs, computers, and phones is the perfect wavelength needed to interfere with hormones released from your brain that are needed for the proper initiation of sleep.[13] If you can't live without your devices before bed, use apps and programs like Night Shift (iOS), f.lux (Windows), and Twilight (Android). These programs and settings reduce and remove the amount of blue light emitted from your devices, theoretically attenuating the damage they would otherwise be doing to your brain and sleep/wake cycle.

## 5. Turn Off the Lights

As the great 1970s soul legend Teddy Pendergrass once crooned, "Turn off the lights." Your brain releases compounds in response to darkness. Lights in your room can interfere with natural processes that occur to get you to sleep and to help you stay asleep. Do an audit of your bedroom at night, ensuring that computer lights, alarm clock lights, and nightlights in the main area where you sleep are *off*—so that they can't negatively impact the quality of your sleep or your ability to stay that way.

## 6. Stay Cool

Because your body doesn't regulate its own temperature during deep sleep, being in a cool room allows you to stay in these restful stages longer. Aim to keep your bedroom between 60° and 67°F degrees. If the temperature fluctuates too much while you're in deep sleep, your body will break out of that phase of sleep so that it can better regulate your body temperature. You need lots of deep physically and mentally restorative sleep, so keep your room cool and consistent to optimize your sleep quality.

## 7. Relax and Stretch

If you find that you're having trouble winding down and relaxing before bed, take 5 to 8 minutes to engage in a simple static stretching routine, holding each stretch for 30 seconds. Despite what most people think, stretching is not an effective strategy for increasing flexibility or getting you ready for a workout, but it is a great way to stimulate your parasympathetic nervous system. This is the "rest and digest" part of your nervous system. Activating your parasympathetic nervous system at bedtime will encourage relaxation and help you get to sleep more efficiently.

## 8. Play Dead

If you ignore all of the sleep advice in this section, just don't ignore this tip. In yoga, there's a pose called corpse pose. The corpse pose should be your final activity before nodding off to sleep. I'm definitely not a yogi, but this is so simple and effective that it's a must-do for great sleep. No yoga training required.

Lie on your bed on your back with your arms straight but slightly away from your sides, palms facing up. Your feet should be 1 to 2 feet apart. Slowly take a deep diaphragmatic breath through your nose and then exhale through loosely pursed lips. The emphasis of your breath needs to be on the prolonged exhalation. When you take a long exhalation, your parasympathetic nervous system is stimulated. This slows your heart rate, reduces your blood pressure, and enhances your overall ability to relax.

Research shows that just 5 minutes of deep breathing like this can significantly lower your heart rate and blood pressure and affect how quickly you fall asleep.

## 9. Build in Catch-Up Sleep

Even if you have the best intentions for getting adequate quality sleep, your lifestyle may not always permit this. Family and work demands on your time can intensify in spurts, leaving you with no choice but to sleep less. The good news is that all is not lost during these times, as you can catch up on lost sleep and correct some of the negative metabolic consequences that we have been discussing. A 2015 study, published in *Clinical Endocrinology*, found that when sleep-restricted men were able to catch up on sleep over the weekend, leptin, testosterone, and other hormones related to blood sugar management all improved.[14] If you're embarking on the MetaShred Diet during a crazy time in your life, and adequate sleep during the week isn't a viable option, make sure to block out time during your weekend to catch up on the lost sleep from the week.

I want to leave you with one last research study to bring home the gravity of good sleep for fat loss. The title of the article actually says it all: "Insufficient Sleep Undermines Dietary Efforts to Reduce Adiposity."[15] You read this correctly. Researchers from the University of Chicago found that insufficient sleep undermined their study participants' fat-loss dieting efforts. In this small clinical trial, participants lost both significantly less fat and more muscle when they got 5.5 hours of sleep a night compared to 8.5 hours.

There's nothing worse than wasted effort. If you're going to do all the work of making sure that you eat the right meals, in the right amounts, at the right times, it would be a shame to have insufficient sleep be the factor that hindered your fat-loss results.

## Stress, Willpower, and Weight Loss

I used to have a running joke with my training partner that he wasn't allowed to talk to me when my heart rate was above 165 beats per minute. The reason: The physiological stress that comes with your heart beating that fast makes it nearly impossible to think logically or intelligently enough to answer any questions.

This is a great example of how the biology of stress and the biology of self-control can't coexist. Self-control requires logical, thoughtful actions, while stress depends on frantic, quick, and often scattered responses. This can be stress from anything—work, life, exercise, whatever.

How successfully you are able to manage and navigate the stress in your life, both ongoing and in-the-moment stressors, will be a major determinant in how successful you are with the MetaShred Diet. It'll also be a key in how well you maintain those fat-loss results in the future.

Nutritional science greatly underestimates and underappreciates the impact that stress has on your eating habits and food choices. Over the years, I've observed in my clients the three most common times during the day where stress negatively impacts nutrition, mainly through snacking to cope with stress.

1. **Midafternoon, or about 2 to 2.5 hours after lunch.** This is when people get hit with a combination of cumulative stress from the day as well as sleep pressure.

The solution is often to reach for something sugary for a boost in energy and coping skills.

2. **After getting home from work, but before dinner.** For many people, this is the first time of the day when they can come up for air from the workday and realize the tension that they've been holding. Combine this with readily available foods, either from the snack cupboard or in preparation for dinner, and you have a recipe for disaster.

3. **After dinner.** This is generally the largest time for unregulated and unaccounted for snacking and calories. It's most likely a combination of TV watching-induced snacking and the further comfort of snacking for coping with stress, or just eating due to boredom.

Unregulated snacking during any or all of these times will easily completely derail your MetaShred Diet efforts, so it's important to gain awareness about which parts of the day you're stressed the most and which parts of the day you're most likely to have the urge to snack. To help you, I've developed several strategies for managing stress-induced nutritional crises, which I'll cover throughout this chapter.

## Get Your Stress Vaccine Regularly

The good news about stress is that a lot of stress is relative. Knowing this gives you a keen advantage. That's because it allows you to manipulate the stress system in your body in order to inoculate yourself to stressors that would otherwise derail your fat-loss efforts.

You can vaccinate yourself against many stressors by practicing a concept developed by psychologist Donald Meichenbaum, PhD, the father of cognitive-behavior therapy. But let me start with a couple of anecdotes to the set the stage.

A mentor of mine laughs when she tells the story of how stressed she was with her first job out of graduate school. At the end of the week, she would have as many as eight unanswered voicemails to deal with. (This was before cell phones and e-mail.) She now manages multiple projects and people across the country, expertly managing her never-ending e-mail inbox, mainly from her cell phone while she is on the go. Now, it's hard for her to imagine that at one time, an answering machine with eight unanswered messages used to stress her out!

Likewise, my wife and I laugh about how *busy* and stressed out we were when we first got married and I was in graduate school. Our mornings were frantic as we tried to get her off to work, get me to the general clinical research center on time, and also somehow get the dog walked. That's compared to now, where we need to pack lunches and get three little kids off to school—with a toddler doing his best to sabotage the process—in addition to each of our morning responsibilities. It's humorous to look at how the mornings used to stress us out!

These are two living examples of stress inoculation training. At its most basic level, stress inoculation training involves progressively exposing yourself to a stressor or stressful situation, until that situation or stressor is no longer stressful.

When you receive a vaccine, you're getting a limited dose of a virus that your body will then combat and build a greater immunity to. This is similar to a concept in biology called hormesis, in which an organism is exposed to a small amount of toxin, and it yields a positive response, but a larger dose yields a negative response.

I'm sure that thinking back on your life, you too will have stories of situations and times where you felt like you were operating under extreme stress. But now, looking back on it, those situations would seem like a cakewalk.

Much of the combat training our military—especially special forces—goes through is grounded in stress inoculation training theory. They make the training and practice so realistic and stressful that the soldiers acclimate to operating under those conditions, so that when the stress of combat happens, they're able to execute the objectives.

When you look at stress this way, you can see that it's very relative and not an absolute thing. What stressed you out 5 to 10 years ago doesn't even make you blink now. What stresses you out now probably wouldn't make an army ranger blink. (Unless you are, in fact, an army ranger reading this; thank you for your service.) This is empowering because whatever is stressing you out now and causing you to make food decisions that you don't really want to make can be trained for and adapted to, so that you can more easily deal with the situation.

## Inoculate Yourself in 3 Steps

We're going to look at stress inoculation training through the lens of stressors in your life that will derail you from the MetaShred Diet. We'll examine three components of stress inoculation training and how they fit into your life, and then we'll go over different strategies for you to plug into the steps.

In practice, stress inoculation training is very flexible, not dogmatic. So when reading the section that follows, keep your focus on the big picture concepts and how you can apply them specifically to yourself and your life.

### Step 1: Education

During this phase of stress inoculation training, you educate yourself about the stressors in your life and how you respond to them. This is as much education as it is assessment. Here are some questions to ask yourself:

■ Do you find yourself struggling with your diet at the three high-stress or let-down times—midafternoon, before dinner, and after dinner—like many of my clients?

■ How do you cope with those moments?

■ Does your response to these times eat away at your ideal behaviors and goals over time?

■ Are there particular triggers when you're experiencing higher levels of stress that cause you to reach for food?

- Are there specific foods that you gravitate toward when you are stressed?
- Do you find that giving in to snacking urges at night has a negative impact on your ability to get up and work out in the morning? Or your ability to have the optimal breakfast that you want to have?

The answers that you provide should help reveal areas in which you could use help managing your stress. Dealing with stress—and your response to it—is often best done when you isolate and break down larger problems into short-term situations, and then create goals for those short-term situations.

For example, "I always overeat at night" doesn't provide much hope for overcoming the problem. It's much more helpful to say, "When I've had an especially hard day at work, I'll often snack on what's around the house after dinner." You've now connected your problem to a specific situation and identified your in-the-moment response. This type of framing provides you with opportunities to solve the short-term situation and thus address the larger problem. In this case, you might:

- Structure your diet so that you have a larger, more-satisfying meal at night
- Move your afternoon snack to after dinner
- Have more optimal snacks in your house
- Remove less optimal snacks from your house

While this is just one example, you can apply this approach to any of the problems you discovered from asking yourself the questions above.

## Step 2: Acquisition

This is the skills acquisition phase. Now that you have identified the stressors and also some solutions, what are actual skills that you need to acquire in order to be better prepared to handle these stressors? In the coming pages, I will outline for you my three go-to techniques that I use with clients: nutrition audibles, surfing the urge, and tactical breathing. You'll be able to apply them to your life right away. I recommend that you practice them whenever possible, as they will become your aces in the hole as you get going with the MetaShred Diet and beyond.

## Step 3: Application

This is where you apply the new skill set that you're about to learn. Anytime you become stressed, you'll actively practice your coping skills and leap over that nutritional land mine that you would have otherwise fallen face-first, mouth-wide-open into.

I want you to look at the three steps of stress inoculation training as a new, overarching philosophy for how you approach and deal with stress in your life, especially as it's related to nutrition and healthy habits. This is not a linear or finite process. It's fluid and ever-changing. But understanding the framework of stress, how it affects you, and your response to it is essential. This understanding will give you the skill sets you need to dominate this area of your life/diet.

As we move on to the nitty-gritty of the three skills you'll need, I want to emphasize that the stress you experience in your life, and your response to it, is normal. This includes the desire to eat high-carbohydrate, high-fat foods. In fact, the cravings for these foods are driven by systems in your body that relieve the stress that you're feeling. Of course, from a weight-loss and health perspective, it's not your best course of action to use food to appease these processes, which is why I'm going to give you alternatives.

We all eat or modify our eating in response to stress at one time or another, and to different degrees. You might not consider yourself a "stress-eater." But upon closer examination, I'm sure you'll find that you have certain eating habits that you've developed in response to stress, or certain food decisions that you make only when you're under stress. This will dictate how much and how often you use the strategies outlined ahead in your life.

## Stress-Fighting Skill 1: Develop Nutrition Audibles

Even if you do your best to vaccinate against the stressors in your life, you're still going to have to deal with stress and how it impacts your diet. The best piece of advice that I have for you is this: Don't make food or health decisions while you're stressed.

In football, quarterbacks have a series of plays that they can call at a moment's notice if they see a big problem coming from the opposition's defense. The quarterback doesn't say, "This doesn't look good, but let's just hike the ball and hope for the best." Instead, he quickly implements a contingency plan, called an audible, and turns a lost play into a potential gain. You need to do the same. Don't freestyle, audible.

The basis of the nutritional audible is solving your problems when you have a clear head. It's really hard to make the *right* nutritional choice in the moment, when you're stressed and tired. It's much easier to know that the decision has been made ahead of time, and you just need to execute the script.

I have a client who usually works late 1 to 2 nights a week. Every night, around 11:00 p.m., she gets the urge to snack. It's probably not a shocking revelation that good snacking rarely happens this late at night. It was no different with my client, as she usually ended up walking down the block and getting a slice of pizza.

We developed two audibles for this situation. The first was to have a Greek yogurt, a small amount of berries, and some almonds in the fridge near her desk. So when she was having trouble fighting the urge, there would be good options conveniently located. The second audible was our "abort plan." If she headed out to get a slice of pizza, it was time to abort the mission. Walk right by the pizza place and go home. Having these two preplanned options has made all the difference in the world with this client's late-night eating habits.

Another way that I like to implement audibles for clients is standard ordering procedures (SOPs). Often, our diet plans can get disrupted due to scheduling changes that are out of our control. SOPs are a small collection of meals that you know you can get just about anywhere and that fit into your diet protocol.

With the franchising of America, you know that the same 5 to 10 restaurants will be available wherever you are. Pick your favorite places, go online, and look at the nutrition facts for meals to determine which items you would order at each place. Select a breakfast, lunch, and dinner option. Then, no matter what happens or where you are, you will be able to execute your SOP and get a *good-enough* meal—all without having much to think about and with no wiggle room to convince yourself otherwise. In the absence of SOPs, it's all too easy to let yourself off the hook "this one time." Be on the offensive, or get sucked into ordering buffalo wings.

SOPs aren't just for ordering out. It's good to have them ready as quick meals at home that you can throw together in 5 to 10 minutes with ingredients you always have on hand. You should also have a SOP shake that's your go-to item in a pinch. With all of the MetaShred recipes provided in this book, you'll have plenty of options with which to put together your SOPs.

Here are two situations in day-to-day life where SOPs are extremely valuable.

## Situation 1: Work Gets in the Way

You have lunch in the fridge at work, but your off-site meeting went over schedule, and you had to run to another meeting across town. This means that you aren't able to get to your office and eat like you had planned. What do you do?

Armed with your SOPs for one to two restaurant franchises in your area, it's easy to select a meal, order, and eat before you head to your next meeting. There are even restaurants with ordering apps now. These apps will allow you to create "favorite meals" with your ordering specs already built in. So you're just a couple of clicks away from an optimal meal. No excuse, just execution.

## Situation 2: Family Life Throws You a Curveball

Perhaps this sounds familiar: One of your children gets sick, and you need to take her to the doctor first thing in the morning. In all the madness, you aren't able to make the frittata that you had planned. What do you do?

In this situation, you can blend up a quick smoothie that is on your at-home SOP list. My go-to smoothie is the MetaShred Smoothie (see page 174). If you don't have time to whip one up, you then could refer to your SOP list for drive-thru breakfast places and grab a good-enough meal somewhere along the way.

With nutritional audibles and SOPs, the main point is to reduce the mental friction of getting a healthy meal. There's usually zero friction for getting unhealthy foods, and it's the friction of getting optimal meals that makes people toss up their hands in defeat.

## Stress-Fighting Skill 2: Surf the Urge

One of my favorite in-the-moment stress-management strategies is one that I've borrowed from an addiction treatment therapy developed by the late, great Alan Marlatt, PhD, the former director of Addictive Behaviors Research Center at the University of Washington. I always tell clients that if this can help stop an alcoholic from pouring a drink or a former smoker from lighting up, it can help keep you from raiding the mini-fridge at the end of the hall.

Dr. Marlatt would explain to his patients that cravings and urges are not something that we can get rid of, but instead, they're always going to be there. And since we have to live with them, we also need to learn to effectively deal with them.

Food cravings are no different. If you have a sweet tooth, you're never going to "unsweeten" your tooth. This is an important piece to understand, as I have had many clients who get frustrated with their food cravings—annoyed that they can't get rid of them. It's a fruitless pursuit. So let's move on and get productive by developing strategies to work through them without giving in to them.

"Surfing the urge" is one such strategy. The origins of it are rooted in an interaction that Dr. Marlatt had with a patient, who happened to be a surfer and wanted to quit smoking. While surfing the urge was developed as an intervention for helping people to quit smoking, you will quickly see the parallels with food cravings.

The surfer expressed frustration that once he got the urge to smoke, he could only last 45 minutes or so before lighting up. The more he tried to fight it, the stronger and stronger the urge would become. Dr. Marlett encouraged the surfer to envision his urge to smoke as a wave approaching the shore. The wave grows and grows, getting stronger and stronger, but then when it gets to shore, the wave subsides.

His point: Urges don't continue to get stronger and stronger until you give in; it just seems that way. They all dissipate, like waves.

Dr. Marlett would have his patients slow down their breathing and envision themselves riding the "urge wave" until it subsided. Sure, you'll metaphorically crash on a couple of waves and give in to your craving; just keep working at it. Over time, the urge waves will get farther and farther apart, and you'll get better and better at riding them. Dr. Marlett's surfer patient used this exercise to quit smoking entirely after just 5 weeks of being introduced to the concept.

The truth is, even if you apply all of the strategies in this book, you're going to be hungry at times, and you're going to crave foods. Part of the problem for the rapid fat-loss dieter is that the MetaShred Diet involves intensifying regular fat-loss strategies. So, at times, you'll rely more heavily on self-control than you would in a more traditional fat-loss diet. When you find yourself in these situations, surf the urge! Slow down your breathing a little and feel the urge. Don't get mad that you have the desire, but instead acknowledge it and try to ride it out until it dissipates. In addition to surfing the urge, you can also use tactical breathing.

## Stress-Fighting Skill 3: Tactical Breathing

As we talked about when discussing sleep, staying properly relaxed can be challenging when in the throes of rapid fat-loss dieting. This is especially true when you compound it with the additional normal work and family stress. For this reason, I insist that all of my clients practice some sort of daily deliberate stress reduction (DSR). Every day, you need to purposefully do something that helps you manage your stress load. It's like a daily closet cleaning for your brain. I notice a marked difference in the fat-loss success of clients who are committed to daily DSR and those who are not.

Mindfulness is currently the gold rush for health and weight loss. It seems like it's being pushed as the cure-all for every health ill, from fat loss to heart disease. I don't see mindfulness as a cure-all, but it is a useful tool. If you want to use mindfulness meditation as your daily DSR, that's great. It's my tool of choice as well. There are a handful of apps that are great for guided meditations. Headspace is currently the most popular among my clients, but you can also keep it very simple and just count your breaths.

My primary method of DSR is a simple meditation that uses "tactical breathing." Dave Grossman, a retired lieutenant colonel and US army ranger, put tactical breathing in the forefront of stress management for first responders and military personnel when he cowrote about it in the book, *On Combat: The Psychology and Physiology of Deadly Conflict in War and in Peace.*

The primary purpose of tactical breathing is to slow your breathing rate—down to about four breaths per minute—to reign in your fight-or-flight response. This slow, methodical breathing stimulates your parasympathetic nervous system, leaving you calm and relaxed; as Grossman writes, "[it is used] to bathe yourself with a sense of calm and control."

I use this in two different ways: daily meditation and SOS breathing.

## Daily Meditation

Before my day gets going, I sit in a chair with a straight back with my hands on my lap, or I kneel on my meditation bench, and breathe. Here's what to do.

With your eyes closed, breathe in through your nose as you count to four. When you breathe in, breathe into your stomach, not into your chest. One way to know if you're doing it right: Your shoulders shouldn't shrug up and your neck muscles should stay relaxed. As you breathe into your stomach, don't let your belly just flop out as your abdomen fills with oxygen. Instead provide a little resistance with your ab muscles. This forces your midsection to expand sideways and even backward. In fact, if you're really getting it, you should feel a little stretch in your lower back muscles as the air fills your abdominal cavity.

Once you have inhaled for a slow four count, hold your breath for another four count. Then, gently contract your abs, drawing in your stomach, and squeeze out the air that you have just inhaled—exhaling for a slow four count through lightly pursed lips. Push out all the air that you can. Then hold that exhaled position, with your lungs empty, for another slow four count. That's one set of tactical breathing. Simply focus on the numbers and the sequence while you try to let any other thoughts that enter your mind pass on by.

During my morning meditation, I will cycle through continuous sets of tactical breathing for 5 to 30 minutes, depending on the time I have and how I'm feeling.

## SOS Breathing

With stress comes bad food decisions. During the MetaShred Diet, you're going to need to buffer the stress of life so that it doesn't have you shutting down a Golden Corral—or, more realistically, eating a bag of tortilla chips and guac washed down with three Coronas, when you were scheduled to have a small wedge salad and turkey burger.

This is where SOS tactical breathing comes to the rescue. This is more in line with the traditional use of tactical breathing in the military. However, instead of staying calm in the face of gunfire, you're staying calm in the face of a Five Guys double-patty cheese and bacon burger. When you're in the middle of your daily life, you don't have time to sit and get all Zen, but you can pause and complete four to five sets of tactical breathing. That's less than 90 seconds of effort, but it can help zero out the stress response that was going to derail your diet.

## More Ways to Fight Stress

If meditation isn't your thing, that's fine. Go for a walk at lunch or after dinner (without your phone). Cooking can also be a source of stress reduction, as the detailed nature and the creation of quality meals can be very rewarding. More recently, coloring books for adults have become an extremely popular method for de-stressing. Another favorite DSR practice of mine, and also that of *South Park* creator Trey Parker, is building with Legos.

Pick whatever you enjoy. It doesn't need to be the same thing every day, as long as it fits these criteria.

1. **You must check out.** A key to successful DSR practices is checking out and powering down. Turn off your phone and get away from your computer. If you can, get outside. Being outside is even better, as the stress-reduction benefits of being in nature are well-documented. This helps break the pattern of your day and the stress associated with it.

2. **You must focus.** All good DSR practices require your focus. By focusing on the task at hand, you're not focusing on everything else in your life. Focus on your next breath,

## L-THEANINE: A STRESS-RELIEF SAVIOR?

L-Theanine is a unique amino acid analog found in tea. In the late 1940s, it was discovered as a component of green tea.

L-Theanine works in concert with caffeine to enhance mood, working memory, and cognition. My clients love L-Theanine, as it takes the edge off caffeine, allowing them to get the performance benefits of caffeine without the jitters usually associated with high levels of caffeine consumption.

It may also be able to help lower anxiety and aid in enhancing sleep by increasing alpha waves in your brain. Alpha waves are the predominant brain waves present during meditation and daydreaming. They're also associated with a relaxed mental state. One of the best characteristics of L-Theanine is that it's relaxing but not sedating.

Both regular green tea and matcha—powdered green tea, made from tea leaves grown in the shade—have high levels of L-Theanine. Black tea is also a significant source of L-Theanine.

However, to reap measurable benefits from L-Theanine, supplementation is warranted. That's because L-Theanine levels in tea can range from 5 to 25 milligrams per cup, while research shows that you need a dose of 100 to 200 milligrams to benefit fully.

mincing the garlic just right, or how the blue flat Lego piece fits just right into the structure you're building. If you're at a mental impasse on a project or area in your life, you'll find that shifting your focus to something else will become your secret weapon to de-stressing and overcoming a mental block. Neuroscience research clearly shows that thinking about something other than a problem—instead of thinking *harder* about a problem—is the key to finding a solution.[16]

3. **You must enjoy it.** Your DSR should be something that you look forward to doing, as it's optimizing your physiology, making your fat loss more effective, and, hopefully, making *you* more effective in your day-to-day life. This is why it's important to find something that you enjoy. If you pick mindfulness meditation and find that you're struggling, that's fine! Mindfulness research shows that you don't need to be *good* at meditation. It's through the practice of mindfulness meditation itself that allows you to reap the benefits.

These approaches will help empower you to attack life's stressors head-on. This way, you won't be a victim to limited willpower. Instead, you'll feel as if you're prepared to handle food in any stressful situation or whenever you're faced with intense food cravings.

Be proactive with your stress management. Dedicate yourself to daily DSR even if it's for just 5 minutes. It'll pay off; it always does. Your weight loss will improve and, as a side benefit, it's great for your longevity.

## Build a Better Fat-Loss Culture

I cringe a little using the word *culture* because it has become such a buzzword in business that it's lost a lot of its impact. But culture is the best way to describe what you need to foster.

Making healthy choices by choosing to eat a little less and move more so that you can hit your fat-loss targets is tough. Like, the-world-is-out-to-sabotage-you-and-see-you-fail tough. Don't try to go this alone. Over the years, the clients of mine who have a supportive fat-loss culture around them get the best results.

You need to create and foster a culture of healthy habits so that you aren't making healthy decisions because you're forcing them upon yourself, but because that's what you want to do. Here are two examples to illustrate my point.

My kids eat fruits and vegetables at every meal, and when they snack on baby carrots and red pepper strips during the day, they say things like, "Mmmm, that's delicious!" They eat broccoli and peas by the handful. Literally, it's a struggle to get my oldest son to use a spoon. They eat this way because that's just how we eat (the vegetable part, not the spoonless part).

Eating vegetables has never been an issue for them, because those are the foods that we eat. Fruits and vegetables were never singled out as foods that we don't really want to eat but do because we have to. We just eat them; that's the culture at our house.

I used to do nutrition consulting out of a gym in Manhattan called PEAK Performance. One of the things that I loved about visiting PEAK was the food culture there. All of the trainers generally ate really well, as that was the culture. If you came to the gym with unhealthy food, you'd get made fun of in a playful but positive way. However, that social pressure was enough to make you want to clean up your act and step up your food game.

Sometimes, you need that. Sometimes, when you're tired and your guard is down, you need the added peer pressure to stay the course and order your burger without the bun. And to substitute the fries for vegetables, instead of eating the menu item as it comes.

I give all of my clients a social support/culture questionnaire to assess the kind of environment in which they're executing their diet and exercise program.

- Is it a supportive one? Adversarial one?
- What is the culture of your social circle like?

When you make a healthy choice on a menu or request a meal be prepared a certain way—so that you can stick to your diet plan—is that supported by your peers? Or is it met with undermining comments about how you are "always eating healthy" or "Why don't you just enjoy yourself a little?" Even if your friends are joking—I don't think most people say those things to be overtly malicious—it wears on you.

It isn't all on your friends. You need to communicate with them what you're doing, why you're doing it, and what you need from them. If you've never communicated to your friends about your MetaShred fat-loss goals—and how you would like their support—how can you fault them for not supporting you?

You don't need to have a sit-down kumbaya diet/emotions session with them, but you can take 5 minutes to let them know about what you're doing with MetaShred. You can tell them how you're excited about it and what the sacrifices you're going to have to start making will be. It's much easier to let your friends know ahead of time that you won't be your normal five-beer self at the weekly Friday happy hour than it is telling them at the bar while your buddy slams a cold one into your hand.

If your social group doesn't have a good fat-loss culture, that doesn't mean you need to dump those friends for new ones. But it does mean that you should seek out like-minded people who can support you on your journey. And in turn, you can support them.

Find someone you can share your favorite MetaShred recipe with or someone who can be an accountability partner for your MetaShred Diet adherence. Even if there isn't a person in your immediate physical social circle, look online. Research on effective online weight-loss programs shows that personal accountability and interaction is consistently the determining factor in one's long-term success.[17]

Use the hashtag #metashred on Instagram, Twitter, or your favorite social platform to get virtually connected with people from all over the place who, like you, have made the commitment to the MetaShred way of life. The point about culture is that you want to immerse yourself in a culture where the healthy habits that you hold important are the norm. This is key for getting the most out of MetaShred but also for maintaining a lean body for the long haul.

## Get a Chip on Your Shoulder

I want to close out this chapter with a controversial discussion on mind-set. I debated the inclusion of this section in the book, but it's something that I discuss with all of my clients at one time or another, so I think it's important to discuss with you.

Get a chip on your shoulder about your ability to take control of your diet and your ability to execute. A sense of lack of control is the worst thing. This is a common characteristic among chronically overweight people with whom I have worked. So when you get control and are working your plan, feel good about it!

After all, nearly 70 percent of the U.S. population is overweight or obese. You're succeeding against all odds!

Against 99.8 percent of all food marketing.

Against every gadget that makes life "easier" so that you can move and do less.

Against all of the thoughts flying in and out of your mind each day, telling you to skip the gym or to have the leftover pancakes on your kid's plate!

Foster a little feeling of pride in your daily efforts and execution. This doesn't *need* to have negative connotations. It doesn't mean that you're putting others and their dietary foils down. There's enough of that on the Internet, and it's shameful.

But I do want you to recognize that you are doing something great, something that pretty much everyone wants to do but hasn't been able to do consistently. Compliance to dietary plans is the elephant in the room when it comes to failed research studies.

For instance, in an editorial in the *American Journal of Clinical Nutrition*—the undisputed top clinical nutrition research journal in the world—Walter Willett, MD, DrPH, of Harvard T. H. Chan School of Public Health, wrote about how two separate multiyear, multimillion dollar research trials both failed to test the initial research questions due to the inability of study participants to adhere to the study protocols.

The MetaShred Diet is all about compliance. In Chapters 6 and 7, I'm going to spell out for you, in more detail than you can imagine, exactly what you need to eat and exactly when you need to eat it. I'm removing the mystery from rapid fat loss—but the hard part is *doing it,* day in and day out.

It's the mental stuff that will make or break your progress. By the time you get to the end of this book, you will know exactly how to execute an effective rapid fat-loss diet. The only thing left for you to do is set your mind to unwavering execution.

As you start this program, and as you execute day after day, give yourself credit for raging against the obesogenic machine of our daily lives, doing what most people won't. Use that good feeling—that chip on your shoulder—to fuel your persistence even more.

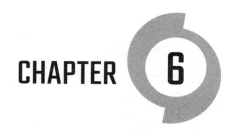

CHAPTER **6**

# The MetaShred Diet: Get Started

've put meal plans together for you that you can follow to a T, or you can build your own meal plan from the recipes and meal templates provided. When you're picking your meal plan, I would like for you to consider two things: preference and execution.

Variety in your diet is generally overrated and misunderstood. People often hear that they need to eat a variety of foods and then set out to create a dish of the week around each vegetable in the produce section.

The excerpt that follows, from the 1995 Dietary Guidelines for Americans, succinctly describes the goal of dietary variety: "Foods contain combinations of nutrients and other healthful substances. No single food can supply all nutrients in the amounts you need. For example, oranges provide vitamin C but no vitamin $B_{12}$; cheese provides vitamin $B_{12}$ but no vitamin C. To make sure you get all of the nutrients and other substances needed for health, choose the recommended number of daily servings from each of the five major food groups displayed in the Food Guide Pyramid."[1]

As this excerpt points out, diet variety is about making sure you eat a great enough variety of foods to meet your vitamin and mineral needs. If you like eating oranges, then eat them. You don't need to eat an orange one day, an apple the next, and a kiwifruit the next, all in the name of dietary variety. They all have vitamin C; just eat the one you like.

The problem with pursuing a diet with a lot of variety is that more variety means more things to remember, purchase, prepare, and eat—making a more complicated diet. The more complicated your diet is, the harder it is to execute and thus adhere to.

Diet adherence is your number one objective. The simpler your food logistics, the better your adherence will be.

I've noticed over the years that clients ask for variety in their diets. They want a large variety of meals choose from so that they don't get bored. But, when it comes down to it, people really just want to eat the same thing over and over. It's this repetition of meals that leads to the greatest success. This is the variety paradox.

On the surface, you may feel the desire to have more options, but the more options you have for meals, the harder it will be for you to execute your diet on a day-to-day basis. When building your MetaShred Diet, pick enough of a variety that you won't be bored with the monotony of the diet, but not so many different meals that the variety becomes a burden.

## What about Those Vitamins and Minerals?

If you eat a well-balanced diet with a variety of fruits, vegetables, lean proteins, and some starches and grains—and let your level of diet variety be based on personal preference and food logistics—do you still get all of your vitamins and minerals?

The uncomfortable truth that most nutritionists or popular diet authors don't want to tell you is that their diets are not 100 percent nutritionally adequate. A 2010 nutritional analysis from the diets used in the A to Z Study—a 12-month weight-loss study that pitted the Atkins, Ornish, Zone, and LEARN diets against each other—found that all of the diets put people at risk for vitamin and mineral inadequacy for a handful of different nutrients. Each diet emphasized or restricted certain types of foods, so the inadequate nutrients varied from diet to diet. But even the LEARN diet, which was modeled after the *Dietary Guidelines for Americans*, left study participants needing more vitamin E, thiamine, and magnesium.[2]

The reason for this is twofold. First, it's really hard, maybe impossible, to create a diet that's easy to execute for people on a daily basis and that also meets 100 percent of the Recommended Dietary Allowance (RDA) for essential vitamins and minerals. Second, as you eat less food—as you would on any calorie-restricted diet—you have fewer opportunities to get all of the vitamins and minerals that you need.

There's a silver lining here, though. The A to Z Study researchers did conclude, "There may be a micronutrient advantage to diets providing moderately low carbohydrate amounts and diets that contain nutrient-dense foods." What they were saying is that when you eat a lower-carbohydrate diet, you end up eating more vegetables—especially the green and leafy kind. These kinds of foods contain more concentrated levels of vitamins and minerals, particularly key minerals like potassium, which

# VITAMIN D: THE HEALTH HERO

Vitamin D is known as the sunshine vitamin, since your body can convert sunlight into vitamin D. Unfortunately, because of most people's indoor-office lifestyle, they don't get enough time in the sun, with enough skin exposed, to meet their needs. I have a fair amount of clients in California, and even most of them need to supplement with vitamin D.

Vitamin D is one of the hottest vitamins in nutrition research right now. Initially, its claim to fame was for its role in bone health, but more and more research is highlighting its potential importance in a variety of areas of health such as:

- Cancer-risk reduction (colon, prostate, and breast cancers)

- Diabetes
- High blood pressure
- Atopic dermatitis
- Arthritis
- Asthma
- Inflammatory bowel disease
- Acute respiratory infections

Vitamin D is a major player in your health, and according to the Institute of Medicine, supplementation with up to 4,000 IU is safe for the general public. One important note: It's a fat-soluble vitamin (as are vitamins A, E, and K). This means that you should take your vitamin D supplement with a meal, as dietary fat is needed to allow your body to access and use the vitamin.

most people come up drastically short in. This is what I have you do with the MetaShred Diet.

In the name of helping you to get not just your *best* body but also your *healthiest* body, I've taken the nutritional rigor of the MetaShred Diet one step further. I ran numerous diet plan simulations to analyze the vitamin and mineral landscape of the MetaShred Diet based on the recipes that I've created for you. Unfortunately, the full nutrition facts for all vitamins and minerals are not available for every food. This creates unaccounted-for error in the analysis, making some nutrients appear inadequate when, in reality, you're actually getting adequate amounts. However, my analysis shows that the following vitamins and minerals consistently miss hitting 100 percent of the RDA across the different MetaDiet levels.

- Thiamine
- Riboflavin
- Pantothenic acid
- Folate
- Vitamin D
- Vitamin E
- Calcium
- Magnesium
- Copper
- Iron
- Zinc
- Vitamin $B_{12}$

Nutrients like thiamine, riboflavin, and pantothenic acid are all B vitamins found primarily in grains, which the MetaShred Diet is low in. So missing the mark for those nutrients isn't surprising.

I was also not surprised to see vitamin D and magnesium show up as inadequate in the analysis, as I haven't had a client in almost 10 years who hasn't benefited from more magnesium and vitamin D. However, the levels of nutrient inadequacy for any of the nutrients listed are so small that they can easily be eradicated by taking a simple once-daily multivitamin with a meal. Women should take the women's version or women's formulation, as it will contain more calcium and iron.

If you want to take your vitamin and mineral supplementation one step further—and I recommend that you do—take an additional 3,000 IU of vitamin D with a meal and 200

## MAGNESIUM: THE MIRACLE MINERAL

Magnesium is the fourth most abundant mineral in the body and is a required component for more than 300 different reactions in your body. Magnesium is a physiological superstar, as it has a role in regulating blood sugar, energy metabolism, and blood pressure.

However, your body doesn't do the best job of holding on to magnesium—especially when you exercise. Blood magnesium levels can decrease as much as 5 percent from just walking on a treadmill for 90 minutes at 3 miles per hour. A 2006 study with female tennis players found that every player enrolled in the study failed to meet daily magnesium requirements.[3]

Magnesium is of the utmost importance when you're active, since sweating can lead to mineral depletion. Research studies have gone on to show that supplementing with magnesium to ensure optimum levels leads to significant improvements in cardiovascular function during exercise and improved tolerance for exercise during times of inadequate sleep.[4]

Individuals have different tolerances to magnesium, and too much can have you running to the bathroom. Start off your magnesium supplementation with 200 milligrams before bed—it may help with relaxation and help you get to sleep—and move up to 400 milligrams, based on your personal tolerance. I recommend chelated magnesium, which are minerals that have been combined chemically with amino acids to form "complexes." You'll know if it's the right product if it lists magnesium glycinate, magnesium citrate, or magnesium gluconate.

to 400 milligrams of chelated magnesium prior to bed. (See "Vitamin D: The Health Hero," on page 85, and "Magnesium: The Miracle Mineral," above.)

## If It Doesn't Feel Like You're Cheating, You're Not Doing It Right

There's no reason you should eat foods that you don't enjoy. One of my early mentors told me, "Mike, people don't want to eat healthy foods; they want to be told that the foods that they are eating are healthy." This is very sage advice, and I have spent a significant portion of my career trying to come up with healthy versions of foods that my clients enjoy.

I had a client who was a professional basketball player who loved chili-cheese dogs. (Who doesn't, right?) I was able to come up with a healthy version of a chili-cheese dog that fit perfectly into his diet parameters. He even told me that he didn't want to eat it in front of his teammates, as he didn't want them to think he was cheating on his diet!

Just this year, I helped a friend diet down to 5 percent body fat in time for his 50th birthday. Throughout the 5 months that we worked together on this, he was constantly texting me asking if the recipes I gave him were actually healthy. He said they tasted too good to be good for him. I would say that he had low expectations for fat-loss diet food. And it's true: When he was in college, he competed in a bodybuilding contest and ate orange roughy and broccoli exclusively for 12 weeks leading up to the competition!

The point is: Good food can also be good for you. You just need to put in a little extra work to make sure that the calories are controlled, preparation methods are correct, and the portions are going to be large enough. Historically, delicious foods have relied on the two "flavor crutches": butter and salt. Basically, if you add enough butter and salt to a meal, it's bound to taste good. Add those two ingredients in with ungodly amounts of carbs, and how could the meal not taste delicious?

The MetaShred Diet takes food to a new level by working with the inherent qualities found in foods to bring out their natural flavors—through proper cooking, seasoning, and combining of ingredients. Here's a good example. During Phase 2, one of the lunch/dinner meals that you can have is the Ultimate Steak Dinner (see page 196). On the surface, something called the Ultimate Steak Dinner doesn't sound like a meal that would be on a weight-loss program. But it is, and here's how.

First, you have to pick the right steak. Certain cuts of meat are better grilled/broiled, while others are better braised or slow-cooked. For decades, the only steak you would see in fitness magazines was a grilled flank steak. Due to its high amount of internal connective tissue, grilling, broiling, or searing a plain flank steak will give you an experience similar to eating a rubber hose. It certainly won't seem indulgent. But you can get around this unpleasant eating experience by marinating the steak for several hours or cooking via moist heat, such a slow cooker or Dutch oven.

As you can see, picking the wrong cooking method for a certain piece of meat can make or break how good a meal will taste. For the Ultimate Steak Dinner, I picked sirloin steak for the recipe because it's a lean cut that can be quickly rubbed with spices and grilled, but also because it's a very versatile cut of meat. So you can use it for other meals during the week. This gives you a tasty cut of meat that can be quickly cooked and repurposed for lunch or another dinner.

What really makes this meal the ultimate meal isn't the beef, but the complements to the beef. I'm talking about mushrooms, blue cheese, and soy sauce (used in the quick

## THE WORLD'S MOST DELICIOUS FLAVOR

Growing up, we were all taught the four tastes: sweet, sour, salty, and bitter. Savory was left out. Umami is the savory taste. You may have never heard of umami, but if you know MSG, then you know umami. Despite its food lore, MSG is nothing fancy. As the name monosodium glutamate suggests, MSG is just a single sodium molecule stuck together with the amino acid glutamate. The sodium/salt molecule is present as a molecular scaffolding to secure the glutamate, but it's glutamate that's responsible for all of the taste.

It's the savory taste from glutamate that Kikunae Ikeda, a Japanese scientist, described as umami (translated as "delicious taste") back in 1908—upon doing a chemical analysis of his family's dashi broth in an effort to determine why it was so delicious. It was the kelp (or kombu), which is loaded with umami flavor, that was the driving force behind the great soup.

Foods rich in umami flavor include: tomatoes, cheese (especially aged cheese), mushrooms, beef, fish, soy sauce, fish sauce, cured meats, tofu, kelp, seaweed/nori, and Worcestershire sauce. Your mouth loves umami as noted by the fact that umami tastebuds are found all over your tongue, while tastebuds for all other tastes—for example, salt and sweet—are confined to specific regions of your tongue.

caramelized onions portion of the dish). These three ingredients are rich in the fifth taste, umami (see "The World's Most Delicious Flavor" on page 89).

What's really awesome about umami-rich foods is that their taste and flavor are synergistic. So when you add four umami-rich foods together, you don't get a taste rating of four, but instead, umami taste math is $1 + 1 + 1 + 1 = 15$! For the MetaShred dieter, this taste explosion comes at no extra caloric cost.

There are 54 MetaShred Diet recipes for you to choose from, with meals ranging from a Sloppy Joe Bowl (page 190) to Fat-Loss Shrimp Fajitas (page 161) to the Ultimate Steak Dinner. I'm a lover of great food, and I wouldn't want you to have to eat anything less than great food while on this program.

## You Don't Have to Eat Kale

Pick the meals that you enjoy, and don't force yourself to eat things that you aren't really fond of. No food is so good for you that you should force yourself to eat it. This is a message that not enough people hear.

Last April, I gave a talk to a group of dietitians and fitness professionals in Austin, Texas. After my talk, there was a luncheon where we shared a meal and talked about different aspects of nutrition and working with clients. The conversation found its way to kale, as you might expect when sitting with these types of folks. Out of the nine of us at the table, seven of us admitted that we can't stand kale (myself included). However, all of the dietitians reported having numerous clients who would tell them they were trying to eat healthy and listed kale as proof of their healthy eating.

Let me tell you, kale doesn't make your diet healthy. If you don't like it, don't eat it. Yes, kale has fiber, a variety of vitamins, and some antioxidants that might have cancer-risk-reducing properties. However, there's always an alternative. If you don't like kale, eat broccoli, cabbage, or Brussels sprouts; they're all vegetable cousins of kale and provide many of the same nutritional benefits.

I've designed the MetaShred Diet to have a lot of flexibility so that you aren't force-feeding yourself "healthy" foods that you don't enjoy eating, but instead can eat nutritionally optimized meals that you love.

## The World's Easiest Nutrition Planner: MetaDiet Levels

As I documented earlier in the book, for decades, the math of fat loss was presented as a very simple and straightforward calculation. All you needed to do was use an equation to determine how many calories a person was burning each day and then create a diet that provided fewer calories than that number. Remember: calories in < calories out = weight loss!

While this approach works to some extent, it's far from optimal. It's important to appreciate the fact that determining the appropriate number of calories, protein, carbohydrates, and fats that a person should be eating—in order to lose maximum fat in minimum time—is more of an art than a science. I'm going to show you how the MetaShred Diet can accelerate you to da Vinci status, by the time you get to the end of this chapter, using the most fundamental principle in science. I'm talking so basic that even my 5-year-old knows how to do it.

When developing the MetaShred Diet, I wanted it to be a plug-and-play plan that allows you to easily adjust your food intake for sustained and consistent fat loss, but without counting calories. To do that, I created a system called MetaDiet Levels that does all of the background calculating for you.

There are five MetaDiet Levels—A through F—that you can use during the program. The MetaDiet Levels all follow the same general meal schedule of:

- Breakfast
- Lunch
- Dinner
- Snack
- Postworkout protein shake

## Breakfast, Lunch, and Dinner

For each meal in your plan, you'll see there's a size—large or small—associated with it. When you use the recipes for that meal, simply choose the one that corresponds to your prescribed meal size. The calories have already been factored into your plan. All you have to do is eat.

## Snack

As a reminder, you can have your snack whenever you want during the day. I recommend that you have it between lunch and dinner. This is the time of day when most people have the biggest dip in their energy levels, while also feeling the biggest load of accumulated stress from the day.

## Postworkout Protein

Right after you finish exercising is a special time. Your muscles are primed to soak up carbohydrates, and your body turns its focus toward rebuilding and repairing the muscle that has been damaged during exercise. Research shows that feeding your muscles protein at this time will enhance the signals to your muscles that drive this rebuilding and repair.[5] Take advantage of this unique time in your physiology. You can use the protein supplement of your choice, but please choose a product that fits the general criteria below. Whey protein or a combination of whey and casein proteins are preferred to other protein supplements, due to their high concentration of essential amino acids and high rate of absorption and uptake by the body.

## Protein Powder Characteristics

- 27 to 33 grams of protein
- Less than 3 grams of fat
- Less than 5 grams of carbs

Most commercially available protein powders contain 20 to 25 grams of protein per scoop. So you'll need to use about 1.5 scoops to meet your postworkout protein needs of 30 grams. On days that you don't work out, skip the postworkout protein shake.

# Determine Your MetaDiet Level

To get started, you need to *estimate* how many calories you're currently burning on a daily basis. You'll take that amount of calories and then subtract some—so that you'll be in a calorie deficit—and that'll be your starting point. I put the emphasis on *estimate* because all of the equations we have access to for estimating calorie needs are flawed.

There are four primary equations used to estimate calorie needs:

- Harris-Benedict
- Mifflin-St Jeor
- Owen

- World Health Organization/Food and Agriculture Organization/ United Nations University

A systematic review of the predictive nature of these equations, published in the *Journal of the American Dietetic Association*, concluded that we need to use "judgment regarding when to accept estimated [calorie needs] using predictive equations in any given individual. Indirect calorimetry may be an important tool when, in the judgment of the clinician, the predictive methods fail an individual in a clinically relevant way."[6]

A 2007 study looked at the accuracy of these equations on predicting energy needs for hospital patients.[7] This is probably the easiest group to estimate calories for since they don't move around very much. The authors concluded, "No equation accurately predicted [calorie needs] in most hospitalized patients."

Basically, this means that we shouldn't take any calorie values that we generate as if they were set in stone, but instead use them as a starting point. Then, after 1 to 2 weeks, move to a different MetaDiet Level based on how your body is responding to the program.

This is the approach that I have used for years with clients, and it has never failed me—whether I was applying it to an NBA athlete, model, or middle-school phys ed teacher. I'm going to show you how to apply it to your life and body.

To determine your starting MetaDiet Level, we're going to use the Harris-Benedict equation. This equation was developed and published in 1918 by botanist and biometrician

# FAT-LOSS HORMONES 101

One of the reasons why focusing on calories, and just eating fewer of them, doesn't give you the fat loss you desire is because there are a handful of hormones in your body that regulate your appetite and metabolism, as well as your body's ability to burn fat. These hormones can be activated or deactivated based on the types and amounts of food that you're eating. The MetaShred Diet is geared toward optimizing these hormones in order to maximize your results. Here are the six fat-loss hormones that you need to know about.

### Ghrelin

Ghrelin is your hunger gremlin. It is your only hunger hormone. You read that correctly: You only have one hormone that stimulates your appetite. Ghrelin is produced in your stomach and works on your brain to signal that you are hungry. Reducing calories causes a dose-dependent increase in ghrelin, meaning that the more you reduce your calorie intake, the more ghrelin will be released. This is why it's important to lower your calories enough to initiate fat loss, but not so much that you tip off a negative hormonal cascade. One upside is that intense exercise can decrease ghrelin levels.

### Insulin

Insulin plays a very important role in your body related to recovery and blood sugar regulation. However, when carbohydrate intakes are high and insulin is left to run wild in the body, it can inhibit the breakdown and burning of stored fat. Insulin and carbohydrates are very tightly linked. The more carbohydrates you eat, the more insulin will be released.

To optimize insulin for fat loss, aim to get most of your carbohydrates from vegetables and some fruit. Limit grains and starches to smaller portions directly after exercise.

James Arthur Harris, from the Carnegie Institution of Washington, and his colleague, Francis Gano Benedict. Drs. Harris and Benedict used the biometrical data from 136 men, 103 women, and 94 newborns to create these equations. And now a century later, it still works![8]

Here's the information that you'll need: your age, weight in pounds, and height in inches. The equation is as follows:

### Glucagon

Glucagon is a hormone that acts directly opposite to insulin. While insulin stores carbohydrates and builds fat, glucagon is responsible for breaking down stored carbohydrates and fats, and releasing them so that your body can use them for energy. Eating a protein-rich, low-carbohydrate meal is the best way to maximize glucagon release.

### Leptin

Once thought to be the cure for obesity, leptin is an adipokine—a hormone exclusively released from fat cells. Leptin interacts with your brain to get your body to eat less and burn more calories. The key to maximizing the effect of leptin is to optimize your brain's sensitivity to it. You can do this by getting 7 to 9 hours of sleep per night, eating antioxidant-rich berries and vegetables, and losing weight.

### Adiponectin

Adiponectin is another adipokine. The less fat and more muscle you have, the more adiponectin your fat cells will release. Adiponectin is enhanced with exercise and boosts your muscles' ability to use carbohydrates for energy, slashes your appetite, and enhances the speed in which your body can break down fat. It's my favorite fat-loss hormone.

### CCK

Short for cholecystokinin, this hormone is released from the cells in your intestines whenever you eat protein or fat. But CCK doesn't just stay in your gut. Instead, it communicates with your nervous system to flip the satiety switch, while simultaneously working with your stomach to slow the rate of digestion. The end result is that you feel fuller longer. Take full advantage of CCK by making sure you have protein and fat at every meal.

**Basal Metabolic Rate (BMR) = 66 + (6.2 x weight in pounds) + (12.7 x height in inches) — (6.76 x age in years)**

So if you're a 35-year-old man who weighs 190 pounds and are 5 feet 8 inches tall, you would enter the information as follows:

**BMR = 66 + (6.2 x 190 pounds) + (12.7 x 68 inches) — (6.76 x 35 years)**

That becomes:

**BMR = 66 + 1,178 + 863.6 — 236.6**

This yields a BMR of 1,871 calories (when you round up to a whole number).

Now that you know how many calories it would take to sustain your life if you just laid around all day, you need to add on the calories that you burn from your daily activities. To do this, you will multiply your BMR by an activity factor.

### Activity Factors

- Little to no activity = 1.2
- Mildly active during the week = 1.3
- Moderately active during the week = 1.4
- Extremely active during the week = 1.5

For best results, when determining your activity level, err on the side of underestimating it.

If you work a desk job and hardly move during the day, then you would use the activity factor of 1.2. If you work a desk job but also work out 3 to 4 hours a week, use the activity factor of 1.3. If you deliver packages all day, or work construction or for a moving company, then you would use the activity factor of 1.5. Remember, determining your energy needs is more of an art than a science. Just select an activity factor that you think best suits you and your lifestyle, and don't stress over it. The more weight you have to lose, the more conservative you should be in regard to your activity factor.

The next step is multiplying your BMR by your activity factor to determine your total energy expenditure.

#### BMR x Activity Factor = Total Energy Expenditure

For our sample calculation, we will select "Little to no activity," or 1.2, as our activity factor.

**1,871 x 1.2 = 2,245 calories**

Our sample person would need 2,245 estimated total calories to maintain his body weight.

Since your total energy expenditure is the amount of calories you would need to eat to *maintain* your body weight, you need to make an adjustment for weight loss. To do this, subtract 500 calories.

**Total Energy Expenditure — 500 = Starting Calorie Intake**

Continuing with our sample calculation:

**2,245 — 500 = 1,745 calories**

The last step is to translate your starting calorie intake to the corresponding MetaDiet Level. Once you do that, you can forget all about calories and just follow the simple system I've created for you. Note that the MetaDiet Levels overlap, since as I pointed out before, this is more art than science. So if your calculation is exactly, say, 2,100, you can start with either MetaDiet Level D or E, but choosing Level D will create a greater daily calorie deficit. The MetaDiet Levels were designed to fit easily into your life. I'm not asking you to eat six to eight meals per day. Instead, just eat breakfast, lunch, and dinner, like you normally would. Have a snack in the morning or afternoon, and then, after you work out, have a protein shake mixed using water.

You'll be provided with nutritionally optimized recipes to use as part of the MetaShred Diet. There are 27 recipes for each phase: 6 breakfasts, 12 lunches/dinners, 4 snacks, and 5 shakes. Due to the modular nature of the MetaShred Diet, you're free to mix, match, and repeat any recipe for a given meal throughout the phase. For example, if you love the Pumpkin Pancakes (see page 159) in Phase 1, you can have them for breakfast every day of Phase 1, but not for Phase 2. The shakes can be used in replacement of any meal (breakfast, lunch, or dinner).

# The MetaDiet Matrix

| STARTING CALORIE INTAKE | METADIET LEVEL | MEALS/SNACK TEMPLATE |
|---|---|---|
| <1,500 | A | 3 small meals, 1 serving postworkout protein |
| 1,500–1,700 | B | 1 large meal, 2 small meals, 1 serving postworkout protein |
| 1,700–1,900 | C | 2 small meals, 1 large meal, 1 small snack, 1 serving postworkout protein |
| 1,900–2,100 | D | 2 large meals, 1 small meal, 1 large snack, 1 serving postworkout protein |
| 2,100–2,300 | E | 3 large meals, 1 large snack, 1 serving postworkout protein |
| >2,300 | F | 3 large meals, 1 small meal, 1 serving postworkout protein |

When selecting the recipes that you want to use as part of the program, it's important to pay attention to the portion size—large versus small—that's appropriate for you at a given meal. (Just refer to your MetaDiet Level in "The MetaDiet Matrix" above for this information.)

It's also important that you only consume food per the meals and the above MetaDiet Levels. Specifically, please abstain from calorie-containing drinks—that's all energy drinks, fruit juices, nondiet sodas, sweet teas and coffees, lemonade, sports drinks and alcohol. And please don't add extra sauces—barbecue sauce, ketchup, sweet-and-sour sauce, and so on—to your food. Adding these things will impede your ability to get the most out of the program. If you want to add additional herbs and spices to your meals, by all means add them. Here's a short list of items that you can add to your meals and meal plans.

## Meal Add-Ons/Condiments

- Hot sauce
- Sriracha

- Mustards (not honey mustard)
- Soy sauce
- Salt (sea salt will give you more salt flavor with less sodium)
- Pepper
- Garlic or fermented garlic paste
- Worcestershire sauce
- Dried herbs
- Additional spices
- Fresh basil, rosemary, parsley, and other herbs
- ¼ cup kimchi or sauerkraut

Is there something that you want to add to the MetaShred Diet, but it isn't on this list? Just hit me up on Twitter @mikeroussell using the hashtag #metashred and I'll help you out.

**Approved Drinks**

- Tap or spring water
- Green tea
- Black tea
- Herbal tea
- Seltzer, sparkling water (check the label to ensure it's calorie-free)
- Diet soda
- Black coffee or espresso (zero-calorie sweetener)
- One cup of coffee with one cream/sugar per day

# MetaShred Diet Phases

The MetaShred Diet is broken up into two phases. Phase 1 is 14 days, and Phase 2 is 14 days. During Phase 1, you will eat more carbohydrates. During Phase 2, you will shift some of the calories that you're eating from carbohydrate to fat. We make this carbohydrate-to fat-shift between phases 1 and 2 because we are progressively turning you into a fat-burning machine.

As you transition to a lower calorie intake, the higher carbohydrate level in Phase 1 will give you more readily available energy for your daily activities and exercise program. As you move into Phase 2, your fat intake will increase and your carbohydrate intake will decrease, forcing your body to rely more on fat as fuel. A higher-fat diet will help keep you more satisfied after meals, despite your calorie intake being reduced compared to normal. This carb-to-fat transition will also help optimize hormones—such as insulin and leptin—that are associated with improved fat loss.

## Moving MetaDiet Levels during the Phase Transition

If you would like to accelerate weight loss halfway through the program, you can use this approach: At the end of Phase 1, just before you start Phase 2, move down one MetaDiet Level—for example, from Level D to Level C. However, if you're happy with your rate of weight loss, there's no need to change. You might as well eat more food if you can, right? Again, the goal is to eat as much food as possible while losing as much fat as possible. You don't get extra points for eating less and suffering more. The higher you can keep your calories, the easier your transition to maintenance nutrition will be, and the easier it will be to maintain your fat loss.

## Doing MetaShred Back-to-Back

Before starting the MetaShred Diet, I think it benefits you to decide if you're going to do this program for 28 days, as it has been originally designed, or for 56 days (essentially doing the program two times, back-to-back). My recommendation: If you have the time, double up and go for 56. Not because 28 days isn't wildly effective, but because I find that people consistently underestimate how much weight they have to lose.

You might end the first 28 days 10 pounds lighter and think, "I should go for another 10." Just recently, after a client had reached an all-time low weight, he told me that prior to starting the diet, he would have believed this weight would be unsustainable for him. In fact, he would have thought he would be "too light." But once he achieved the weight, he really wanted to lose another 5 pounds.

So if you're feeling ready for the challenge, sign on for 56 days. Just by the math of doing the program longer, you'll lose more weight. You'll also be giving yourself more time to ingrain the habitual food choices and behaviors that go along with the MetaShred Diet. This will pay you big dividends in the future as you work to maintain your new body weight.

If you decide to do the MetaShred Diet phases back-to-back—creating a 56-day fat-loss diet program—I recommend that you use the Phase 1 meals for 28 days (instead of 14) and the Phase 2 meals for the following 28 days. Assess your progress every 2 weeks, and adjust your MetaDiet Level down, as needed.

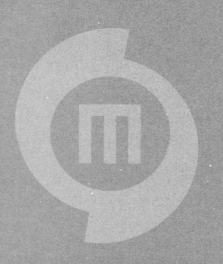

## CHAPTER 7

# MetaShred Meal Plans

'**ve** put together two 28-day meal plans for each MetaDiet level. Phase 1 is your meal plan for the first 14 days; Phase 2 is your meal plan for the last 14 days. If you decide from the beginning to do the program for 56 days, follow Phase 1 for the first 28 days and Phase 2 for the next 28 days. Simply choose your MetaDiet Level based on your calculations on page 98. This allows you to use a meal plan that's customized for your body. You can then use the plan just as provided by eating each meal on the day outlined.

However, if you don't like some of the meals, that's fine. Just sub those out with meals that you would prefer—as long as they're the same size and from the same phase. For instance, you can't sub out a small serving of Fat-Loss Shrimp Fajitas with a large serving of the Open-Face Buffalo Burger and Salad.

| METADIET LEVEL | MEALS/SNACK TEMPLATE |
|---|---|
| A | 3 small meals, 1 serving postworkout protein |
| B | 1 large meal, 2 small meals, 1 serving postworkout protein |
| C | 2 small meals, 1 large meal, 1 small snack, 1 serving postworkout protein |
| D | 2 large meals, 1 small meal, 1 large snack, 1 serving postworkout protein |
| E | 3 large meals, 1 large snack, 1 serving postworkout protein |
| F | 3 large meals, 1 small meal, 1 serving postworkout protein |

Phase 1 = 14 days
Phase 2 = 14 days

# MetaShred Meal-Planning Calendar—MetaDiet Level A; Plan 1

| | SUNDAY | MONDAY | TUESDAY |
|---|---|---|---|
| B: | Small Peanut Butter Cup Parfait | B: Small Pumpkin Pancakes | B: Small Pumpkin Pancakes |
| L: | Small Quick Curry Soup w/ Roasted Chicken | L: Small Quick Curry Soup w/ Roasted Chicken | L: Small Quick Curry Soup w/ Roasted Chicken |
| D: | Small Fenway Park | D: Small Wedge Salad w/ Turkey Burger | D: Small Wedge Salad w/ Turkey Burger |
| S: | 1 Serving Postworkout Protein | S: 1 Serving Postworkout Protein | S: 1 Serving Postworkout Protein |
| B: | Small Chocolate-Cherry Indulgence | B: Small California Scramble | B: Small Pomegranate-Banana Smoothie |
| L: | Small 3-Bean Salad w/ Grilled Garlic Parmesan Chicken | L: Small 3-Bean Salad w/ Grilled Garlic Parmesan Chicken | L: Small Fat-Loss Shrimp Fajitas |
| D: | Small Vietnamese Salad | D: Small Open-Faced Buffalo Burger and Salad | D: Small Open-Faced Buffalo Burger and Salad |
| S: | 1 Serving Postworkout Protein | S: 1 Serving Postworkout Protein | S: 1 Serving Postworkout Protein |

PHASE 1: FAT-LOSS PRIMER

| | WEDNESDAY | | THURSDAY | | FRIDAY | | SATURDAY |
|---|---|---|---|---|---|---|---|
| B: | Small Lumberjack Scramble | B: | Small Peanut Butter Cup Parfait | B: | Small Southwest Eggs Benedict | B: | Small Pomegranate-Banana Smoothie |
| L: | Small Quick Curry Soup w/ Roasted Chicken | L: | Small Quick Curry Soup w/ Roasted Chicken | L: | Small Tomato and Chickpea Salad w/ New York Strip Steak | L: | Small Ultimate Bibb Burger |
| D: | Small Fat-Loss Shrimp Fajitas | D: | Small Kung Pao Chicken | D: | Small Kung Pao Chicken | D: | Small Vietnamese Salad |
| S: | 1 Serving Postworkout Protein | S: | 1 Serving Postworkout Protein | S: | 1 Serving Postworkout Protein | S: | 1 Serving Postworkout Protein |
| B: | Small Peanut Butter Cup Parfait | B: | Small Lumberjack Scramble | B: | Small Southwest Eggs Benedict | B: | Small Superfood Parfait |
| L: | Small Ultimate Bibb Burger | L: | Small Tomato and Chickpea Salad w/ New York Strip Steak | L: | Small Kung Pao Chicken | L: | Small Kung Pao Chicken |
| D: | Small Fenway Park | D: | Small Fat-Loss Shrimp Fajitas | D: | Small Moroccan Chicken w/ Sweet Potato Fries | D: | Small Moroccan Chicken w/ Sweet Potato Fries |
| S: | 1 Serving Postworkout Protein | S: | 1 Serving Postworkout Protein | S: | 1 Serving Postworkout Protein | S: | 1 Serving Postworkout Protein |

# MetaShred Meal-Planning Calendar—MetaDiet Level A; Plan 1

PHASE 2: FAT-LOSS ACCELERATION

| | SUNDAY | | MONDAY | | TUESDAY | |
|---|---|---|---|---|---|---|
| B: | Small Death by Chocolate Smoothie | B: | Small Green Machine Smoothie | B: | Small Coconut-Strawberry Smoothie | |
| L: | Small Herbed Tuna Salad and Avocado Bowl | L: | Small Chicken Caesar Salad | L: | Small Curry Cauliflower w/ Seared Chicken Thighs | |
| D: | Small Turkey Meatball Bowl | D: | Small Turkey Meatball Bowl | D: | Small Turkey Meatball Bowl | |
| S: | 1 Serving Postworkout Protein | S: | 1 Serving Postworkout Protein | S: | 1 Serving Postworkout Protein | |
| B: | Small All-American Breakfast | B: | Small Smooth Herbed Eggs | B: | Small Raspberry-Pistachio Parfait | |
| L: | Small Chef Salad | L: | Small Mediterranean Chicken Lettuce Wraps | L: | Small Mediterranean Chicken Lettuce Wraps | |
| D: | Small Sloppy Joe Bowl | D: | Small Sloppy Joe Bowl | D: | Small Beef Kebabs w/ Tzatziki Sauce | |
| S: | 1 Serving Postworkout Protein | S: | 1 Serving Postworkout Protein | S: | 1 Serving Postworkout Protein | |

| | WEDNESDAY | | THURSDAY | | FRIDAY | | SATURDAY |
|---|---|---|---|---|---|---|---|
| B: | Small Death by Chocolate Smoothie | B: | Small Cheesy Scallion Scramble | B: | Small Smooth Herbed Eggs | B: | Small Raspberry-Pistachio Parfait |
| L: | Small Chef Salad | L: | Small Sloppy Joe Bowl | L: | Small Sloppy Joe Bowl | L: | Small Chicken Caesar Salad |
| D: | Small Turkey Meatball Bowl | D: | Small Curry Cauliflower w/ Seared Chicken Thighs | D: | Small Beef Kebabs w/ Tzatziki Sauce | D: | Small Beef Kebabs w/ Tzatziki Sauce |
| S: | 1 Serving Postworkout Protein | S: | 1 Serving Postworkout Protein | S: | 1 Serving Postworkout Protein | S: | 1 Serving Postworkout Protein |
| B: | Small Crustless Bite-Size Quiche | B: | Small Denver Scramble | B: | Small Coconut-Strawberry Smoothie | B: | Small Cheesy Scallion Scramble |
| L: | Small Pecan-Crusted Salmon w/ Green Beans | L: | Small Grilled Chicken Salad | L: | Small Mediterranean Chicken Lettuce Wraps | L: | Small Mediterranean Chicken Lettuce Wraps |
| D: | Small Beef Kebabs w/ Tzatziki Sauce | D: | Small Ultimate Steak Dinner | D: | Small Pecan-Crusted Salmon w/ Green Beans | D: | Small Herbed Tuna Salad and Avocado Bowl |
| S: | 1 Serving Postworkout Protein | S: | 1 Serving Postworkout Protein | S: | 1 Serving Postworkout Protein | S: | 1 Serving Postworkout Protein |

# MetaShred Meal-Planning Calendar—MetaDiet Level A; Plan 2

<table>
<tr><th></th><th>SUNDAY</th><th>MONDAY</th><th>TUESDAY</th><th></th></tr>
<tr><td rowspan="8">PHASE 1: FAT-LOSS PRIMER</td><td>B: Small MetaShred Smoothie</td><td>B: Small Pumpkin Pancakes</td><td>B: Small Pumpkin Pancakes</td><td></td></tr>
<tr><td>L: Small Fat-Loss Shrimp Fajitas</td><td>L: Small Fat-Loss Shrimp Fajitas</td><td>L: Small Kung Pao Chicken</td><td></td></tr>
<tr><td>D: Small Open-Faced Buffalo Burger and Salad</td><td>D: Small Open-Faced Buffalo Burger and Salad</td><td>D: Small Wedge Salad w/ Turkey Burger</td><td></td></tr>
<tr><td>S: 1 Serving Postworkout Protein</td><td>S: 1 Serving Postworkout Protein</td><td>S: 1 Serving Postworkout Protein</td><td></td></tr>
<tr><td>B: Small Mixed Berry Blast</td><td>B: Small Superfood Parfait</td><td>B: Small California Scramble</td><td></td></tr>
<tr><td>L: Small Spicy Green Chili</td><td>L: Small Spicy Green Chili</td><td>L: Small Ultimate Bibb Burger</td><td></td></tr>
<tr><td>D: Small Tomato and Chickpea Salad w/ New York Strip Steak</td><td>D: Small 3-Bean Salad w/ Grilled Garlic Parmesan Chicken</td><td>D: Small 3-Bean Salad w/ Grilled Garlic Parmesan Chicken</td><td></td></tr>
<tr><td>S: 1 Serving Postworkout Protein</td><td>S: 1 Serving Postworkout Protein</td><td>S: 1 Serving Postworkout Protein</td><td></td></tr>
</table>

| | WEDNESDAY | | THURSDAY | | FRIDAY | | SATURDAY |
|---|---|---|---|---|---|---|---|
| B: | Small Lumberjack Scramble | B: | Small Southwest Eggs Benedict | B: | Small Pomegranate-Banana Smoothie | B: | Small Chocolate-Cherry Indulgence |
| L: | Small Kung Pao Chicken | L: | Small Spicy Green Chili | L: | Small Spicy Green Chili | L: | Small Spicy Green Chili |
| D: | Small Wedge Salad w/ Turkey Burger | D: | Small Wedge Salad w/ Turkey Burger | D: | Small Moroccan Chicken w/ Sweet Potato Fries | D: | Small Moroccan Chicken w/ Sweet Potato Fries |
| S: | 1 Serving Postworkout Protein | S: | 1 Serving Postworkout Protein | S: | 1 Serving Postworkout Protein | S: | 1 Serving Postworkout Protein |
| B: | Small Pumpkin Pancakes | B: | Small Pumpkin Pancakes | B: | Small Chocolate-Cherry Indulgence | B: | Small Lumberjack Scramble |
| L: | Small Vietnamese Salad | L: | Small Vietnamese Salad | L: | Small Moroccan Chicken w/ Sweet Potato Fries | L: | Small Moroccan Chicken w/ Sweet Potato Fries |
| D: | Small Fenway Park | D: | Small Wedge Salad w/ Turkey Burger | D: | Small Wedge Salad w/ Turkey Burger | D: | Small Fat-Loss Shrimp Fajitas |
| S: | 1 Serving Postworkout Protein | S: | 1 Serving Postworkout Protein | S: | 1 Serving Postworkout Protein | S: | 1 Serving Postworkout Protein |

# MetaShred Meal-Planning Calendar—MetaDiet Level A; Plan 2

| | SUNDAY | MONDAY | TUESDAY |
|---|---|---|---|
| **PHASE 2: FAT-LOSS ACCELERATION** | B: Small Creamy Peanut Butter Smoothie | B: Small Coconut-Strawberry Smoothie | B: Small Smooth Herbed Eggs |
| | L: Small Turkey Meatball Bowl | L: Small Turkey Meatball Bowl | L: Small Turkey Meatball Bowl |
| | D: Small Chicken Caesar Salad | D: Small Ultimate Steak Dinner | D: Small Mediterranean Chicken Lettuce Wraps |
| | S: 1 Serving Postworkout Protein | S: 1 Serving Postworkout Protein | S: 1 Serving Postworkout Protein |
| | B: Small Cheesy Scallion Scramble | B: Small Denver Scramble | B: Small All-American Breakfast |
| | L: Small Chef Salad | L: Small Curry Cauliflower w/ Seared Chicken Thighs | L: Small Curry Cauliflower w/ Seared Chicken Thighs |
| | D: Small Pecan-Crusted Salmon w/ Green Beans | D: Small Beef Kebabs w/ Tzatziki Sauce | D: Small Beef Kebabs w/ Tzatziki Sauce |
| | S: 1 Serving Postworkout Protein | S: 1 Serving Postworkout Protein | S: 1 Serving Postworkout Protein |

**B. Breakfast  L. Lunch  D. Dinner  S. Snack**

| | WEDNESDAY | | THURSDAY | | FRIDAY | | SATURDAY |
|---|---|---|---|---|---|---|---|
| B: | Small Raspberry-Pistachio Parfait | B: | Small Crustless Bite-Size Quiche | B: | Small Green Machine Smoothie | B: | Small Banana-Nut Smoothie |
| L: | Small Turkey Meatball Bowl | L: | Small Sloppy Joe Bowl | L: | Small Sloppy Joe Bowl | L: | Small Pecan-Crusted Salmon w/ Green Beans |
| D: | Small Mediterranean Chicken Lettuce Wraps | D: | Small Grilled Chicken Salad | D: | Small Curry Cauliflower w/ Seared Chicken Thighs | D: | Small Ultimate Steak Dinner |
| S: | 1 Serving Postworkout Protein | S: | 1 Serving Postworkout Protein | S: | 1 Serving Postworkout Protein | S: | 1 Serving Postworkout Protein |
| B: | Small Banana-Nut Smoothie | B: | Small Denver Scramble | B: | Small Creamy Peanut Butter Smoothie | B: | Small Coconut-Strawberry Smoothie |
| L: | Small Herbed Tuna Salad and Avocado Bowl | L: | Small Chicken Caesar Salad | L: | Small Chef Salad | L: | Small Curry Cauliflower w/ Seared Chicken Thighs |
| D: | Small Ultimate Steak Dinner | D: | Small Beef Kebabs w/ Tzatziki Sauce | D: | Small Beef Kebabs w/ Tzatziki Sauce | D: | Small Grilled Chicken Salad |
| S: | 1 Serving Postworkout Protein | S: | 1 Serving Postworkout Protein | S: | 1 Serving Postworkout Protein | S: | 1 Serving Postworkout Protein |

## MetaShred Meal-Planning Calendar—MetaDiet Level B; Plan 1

| | SUNDAY | MONDAY | TUESDAY | |
|---|---|---|---|---|
| **PHASE 1: FAT-LOSS PRIMER** | B: Large Southwest Eggs Benedict | B: Small California Scramble | B: Small Superfood Parfait | |
| | L: Small Ultimate Bibb Burger | L: Small Moroccan Chicken w/ Sweet Potato Fries | L: Small 3-Bean Salad w/ Grilled Garlic Parmesan Chicken | |
| | D: Small Moroccan Chicken w/ Sweet Potato Fries | D: Large Kung Pao Chicken | D: Large Kung Pao Chicken | |
| | S: 1 Serving Postworkout Protein | S: 1 Serving Postworkout Protein | S: 1 Serving Postworkout Protein | |
| | B: Large Peanut Butter Cup Parfait | B: Large Southwest Eggs Benedict | B: Small Pomegranate-Banana Smoothie | |
| | L: Small Spicy Green Chili | L: Small Spicy Green Chili | L: Small Spicy Green Chili | |
| | D: Small Wedge Salad w/ Turkey Burger | D: Small Wedge Salad w/ Turkey Burger | D: Large Fenway Park | |
| | S: 1 Serving Postworkout Protein | S: 1 Serving Postworkout Protein | S: 1 Serving Postworkout Protein | |

| | WEDNESDAY | | THURSDAY | | FRIDAY | | SATURDAY |
|---|---|---|---|---|---|---|---|
| B: | Large Pumpkin Pancakes | B: | Large Pumpkin Pancakes | B: | Small Peanut Butter Cup Parfait | B: | Small Lumberjack Scramble |
| L: | Small 3-Bean Salad w/ Grilled Garlic Parmesan Chicken | L: | Small Vietnamese Salad | L: | Large Ultimate Bibb Burger | L: | Small Fat-Loss Shrimp Fajitas |
| D: | Small Tomato and Chickpea Salad w/ New York Strip Steak | D: | Small Fenway Park | D: | Small Vietnamese Salad | D: | Large Ultimate Bibb Burger |
| S: | 1 Serving Postworkout Protein | S: | 1 Serving Postworkout Protein | S: | 1 Serving Postworkout Protein | S: | 1 Serving Postworkout Protein |
| B: | Large Almond Mocha Smoothie Blast | B: | Large MetaShred Smoothie | B: | Small Superfood Parfait | B: | Small Peanut Butter Cup Parfait |
| L: | Small Spicy Green Chili | L: | Small Spicy Green Chili | L: | Large Open-Faced Buffalo Burger and Salad | L: | Large Open Faced Buffalo Burger and Salad |
| D: | Small Kung Pao Chicken | D: | Small Kung Pao Chicken | D: | Small Fat-Loss Shrimp Fajitas | D: | Small Tomato and Chickpea Salad w/ New York Strip Steak |
| S: | 1 Serving Postworkout Protein | S: | 1 Serving Postworkout Protein | S: | 1 Serving Postworkout Protein | S: | 1 Serving Postworkout Protein |

## MetaShred Meal-Planning Calendar—MetaDiet Level B; Plan 1

| | SUNDAY | | MONDAY | | TUESDAY | |
|---|---|---|---|---|---|---|
| B: | Large All-American Breakfast | B: | Small Coconut-Strawberry Smoothie | B: | Small Denver Scramble | |
| L: | Small Chef Salad | L: | Small Pecan-Crusted Salmon w/ Green Beans | L: | Small Pecan-Crusted Salmon w/ Green Beans | |
| D: | Small Ultimate Steak Dinner | D: | Large Beef Kebabs w/ Tzatziki Sauce | D: | Large Beef Kebabs w/ Tzatziki Sauce | |
| S: | 1 Serving Postworkout Protein | S: | 1 Serving Postworkout Protein | S: | 1 Serving Postworkout Protein | |
| B: | Small All-American Breakfast | B: | Small Crustless Bite-Size Quiche | B: | Small Cheesy Scallion Scramble | |
| L: | Large Sloppy Joe Bowl | L: | Small Curry Cauliflower w/ Seared Chicken Thighs | L: | Small Mediterranean Chicken Lettuce Wraps | |
| D: | Small Chef Salad | D: | Large Pecan-Crusted Salmon w/ Green Beans | D: | Large Ultimate Steak Dinner | |
| S: | 1 Serving Postworkout Protein | S: | 1 Serving Postworkout Protein | S: | 1 Serving Postworkout Protein | |

**B. Breakfast    L. Lunch    D. Dinner    S. Snack**

| | WEDNESDAY | THURSDAY | FRIDAY | SATURDAY |
|---|---|---|---|---|
| B: | Small Coconut-Strawberry Smoothie | Small Green Machine Smoothie | Large Banana-Nut Smoothie | Small Raspberry-Pistachio Parfait |
| L: | Large Grilled Chicken Salad | Large Herbed Tuna Salad and Avocado Bowl | Small Chicken Caesar Salad | Large Sloppy Joe Bowl |
| D: | Small Turkey Meatball Bowl | Small Turkey Meatball Bowl | Small Turkey Meatball Bowl | Small Turkey Meatball Bowl |
| S: | 1 Serving Postworkout Protein | 1 Serving Postworkout Protein | 1 Serving Postworkout Protein | 1 Serving Postworkout Protein |
| B: | Large Creamy Peanut Butter Smoothie | Small All-American Breakfast | Small Death by Chocolate Smoothie | Small Smooth Herbed Eggs |
| L: | Small Mediterranean Chicken Lettuce Wraps | Large Pecan-Crusted Salmon w/ Green Beans | Large Chef Salad | Large Grilled Chicken Salad |
| D: | Small Beef Kebabs w/ Tzatziki Sauce | Small Beef Kebabs w/ Tzatziki Sauce | Small Sloppy Joe Bowl | Small Sloppy Joe Bowl |
| S: | 1 Serving Postworkout Protein | 1 Serving Postworkout Protein | 1 Serving Postworkout Protein | 1 Serving Postworkout Protein |

## MetaShred Meal-Planning Calendar—MetaDiet Level B; Plan 2

| | | SUNDAY | | MONDAY | | TUESDAY |
|---|---|---|---|---|---|---|
| **PHASE 1: FAT-LOSS PRIMER** | B: | Small Mixed Berry Blast | B: | Small California Scramble | B: | Large Almond Mocha Smoothie Blast |
| | L: | Small Spicy Green Chili | L: | Small Spicy Green Chili | L: | Small Spicy Green Chili |
| | D: | Large Wedge Salad w/ Turkey Burger | D: | Large Wedge Salad w/ Turkey Burger | D: | Small Vietnamese Salad |
| | S: | 1 Serving Postworkout Protein | S: | 1 Serving Postworkout Protein | S: | 1 Serving Postworkout Protein |
| | B: | Small Pumpkin Pancakes | B: | Small Chocolate-Cherry Indulgence | B: | Small Southwest Eggs Benedict |
| | L: | Small Fat-Loss Shrimp Fajitas | L: | Small Open-Faced Buffalo Burger and Salad | L: | Small Open-Faced Buffalo Burger and Salad |
| | D: | Large 3-Bean Salad w/ Grilled Garlic Parmesan Chicken | D: | Large Kung Pao Chicken | D: | Large Kung Pao Chicken |
| | S: | 1 Serving Postworkout Protein | S: | 1 Serving Postworkout Protein | S: | 1 Serving Postworkout Protein |

| | WEDNESDAY | | THURSDAY | | FRIDAY | | SATURDAY |
|---|---|---|---|---|---|---|---|
| B: | Large Southwest Eggs Benedict | B: | Small Superfood Parfait | B: | Small Lumberjack Scramble | B: | Small Pumpkin Pancakes |
| L: | Small Spicy Green Chili | L: | Small Spicy Green Chili | L: | Large Moroccan Chicken w/ Sweet Potato Fries | L: | Small Fenway Park |
| D: | Small Vietnamese Salad | D: | Large Moroccan Chicken w/ Sweet Potato Fries | D: | Small Ultimate Bibb Burger | D: | Large 3-Bean Salad w/ Grilled Garlic Parmesan Chicken |
| S: | 1 Serving Postworkout Protein | S: | 1 Serving Postworkout Protein | S: | 1 Serving Post workout Protein | S: | 1 Serving Postworkout Protein |
| B: | Small Superfood Parfait | B: | Small Lumberjack Scramble | B: | Small California Scramble | B: | Small Peanut Butter Cup Parfait |
| L: | Large Fat-Loss Shrimp Fajitas | L: | Large Wedge Salad w/ Turkey Burger | L: | Large Wedge Salad w/ Turkey Burger | L: | Large Ultimate Bibb Burger |
| D: | Small Tomato and Chickpea Salad w/ New York Strip Steak | D: | Small Fenway Park | D: | Small Vietnamese Salad | D: | Small Vietnamese Salad |
| S: | 1 Serving Postworkout Protein | S: | 1 Serving Postworkout Protein | S: | 1 Serving Postworkout Protein | S: | 1 Serving Postworkout Protein |

# MetaShred Meal-Planning Calendar—MetaDiet Level B; Plan 2

<table>
<tr><th></th><th>SUNDAY</th><th>MONDAY</th><th>TUESDAY</th></tr>
<tr><td rowspan="4">PHASE 2: FAT-LOSS ACCELERATION</td><td>B: Small Creamy Peanut Butter Smoothie</td><td>B: Small Death By Chocolate Smoothie</td><td>B: Small Coconut-Strawberry Smoothie</td></tr>
<tr><td>L: Large Beef Kebabs w/ Tzatziki Sauce</td><td>L: Large Beef Kebabs w/ Tzatziki Sauce</td><td>L: Large Grilled Chicken Salad</td></tr>
<tr><td>D: Small Herbed Tuna Salad and Avocado Bowl</td><td>D: Small Chef Salad</td><td>D: Small Texas Chili</td></tr>
<tr><td>S: 1 Serving Postworkout Protein</td><td>S: 1 Serving Postworkout Protein</td><td>S: 1 Serving Postworkout Protein</td></tr>
<tr><td>B: Large Crustless Bite-Size Quiche</td><td>B: Small Green Machine Smoothie</td><td>B: Small Denver Scramble</td></tr>
<tr><td>L: Small Chef Salad</td><td>L: Large Sloppy Joe Bowl</td><td>L: Large Sloppy Joe Bowl</td></tr>
<tr><td>D: Small Ultimate Steak Dinner</td><td>D: Small Grilled Chicken Salad</td><td>D: Small Herbed Tuna Salad and Avocado Bowl</td></tr>
<tr><td>S: 1 Serving Postworkout Protein</td><td>S: 1 Serving Postworkout Protein</td><td>S: 1 Serving Postworkout Protein</td></tr>
</table>

**B. Breakfast    L. Lunch    D. Dinner    S. Snack**

| | WEDNESDAY | | THURSDAY | | FRIDAY | | SATURDAY |
|---|---|---|---|---|---|---|---|
| B: | Large Denver Scramble | B: | Small All-American Breakfast | B: | Small Raspberry-Pistachio Parfait | B: | Small Banana-Nut Smoothie |
| L: | Small Chicken Caesar Salad | L: | Large Curry Cauliflower w/ Seared Chicken Thighs | L: | Large Mediterranean Chicken Lettuce Wraps | L: | Large Mediterranean Chicken Lettuce Wraps |
| D: | Small Texas Chili | D: | Small Texas Chili | D: | Small Texas Chili | D: | Small Texas Chili |
| S: | 1 Serving Postworkout Protein | S: | 1 Serving Postworkout Protein | S: | 1 Serving Postworkout Protein | S: | 1 Serving Postworkout Protein |
| B: | Small Crustless Bite-Size Quiche | B: | Small Death by Chocolate Smoothie | B: | Small All-American Breakfast | B: | Small Smooth Herbed Eggs |
| L: | Small Mediterranean Chicken Lettuce Wraps | L: | Small Mediterranean Chicken Lettuce Wraps | L: | Small Pecan-Crusted Salmon w/ Green Beans | L: | Small Curry Cauliflower w/ Seared Chicken Thighs |
| D: | Large Turkey Meatball Bowl | D: | Large Turkey Meatball Bowl | D: | Large Turkey Meatball Bowl | D: | Large Turkey Meatball Bowl |
| S: | 1 Serving Post-workout Protein | S: | 1 Serving Postworkout Protein | S: | 1 Serving Postworkout Protein | S: | 1 Serving Postworkout Protein |

# MetaShred Meal-Planning Calendar—MetaDiet Level C; Plan 1

| | SUNDAY | | MONDAY | | TUESDAY |
|---|---|---|---|---|---|
| B: | Small Southwest Eggs Benedict | B: | Small California Scramble | B: | Large Pumpkin Pancakes |
| L: | Small Tomato and Chickpea Salad w/ New York Strip Steak | L: | Small Fat-Loss Shrimp Fajitas | L: | Small Open-Faced Buffalo Burger and Salad |
| S: | Small Avocado Toast | S: | Small Berries and Cream 2.0 | S: | Small Upgraded Toast and Peanut Butter |
| D: | Large Vietnamese Salad | D: | Large Vietnamese Salad | D: | Small Tomato and Chickpea Salad w/ New York Strip Steak |
| S: | 1 Serving Postworkout Protein | S: | 1 Serving Postworkout Protein | S: | 1 Serving Postworkout Protein |
| B: | Large Almond Mocha Smoothie Blast | B: | Large Superfood Parfait | B: | Small Peanut Butter Cup Parfait |
| L: | Small Kung Pao Chicken | L: | Small Kung Pao Chicken | L: | Large Fat-Loss Shrimp Fajitas |
| S: | Small Upgraded Toast and Peanut Butter | S: | Small Avocado Toast | S: | Small Berries and Cream 2.0 |
| D: | Small Quick Curry Soup with Roasted Chicken | D: | Small Open-Faced Buffalo Burger and Salad | D: | Small Open-Faced Buffalo Burger and Salad |
| S: | 1 Serving Postworkout Protein | S: | 1 Serving Postworkout Protein | S: | 1 Serving Postworkout Protein |

**PHASE I: FAT-LOSS PRIMER**

B. **Breakfast**   L. **Lunch**   D. **Dinner**   S. **Snack**

| | WEDNESDAY | | THURSDAY | | FRIDAY | | SATURDAY |
|---|---|---|---|---|---|---|---|
| B: | Large Pumpkin Pancakes | B: | Small Chocolate-Cherry Indulgence | B: | Small Superfood Parfait | B: | Large California Scramble |
| L: | Small Open-Faced Buffalo Burger and Salad | L: | Large Wedge Salad w/ Turkey Burger | L: | Large Wedge Salad w/ Turkey Burger | L: | Small Fenway Park |
| S: | Small Yogurt and Berries | S: | Small Upgraded Toast and Peanut Butter | S: | Small Yogurt and Berries | S: | Small Upgraded Toast and Peanut Butter |
| D: | Small Quick Curry Soup with Roasted Chicken | D: | Small Quick Curry Soup with Roasted Chicken | D: | Small Quick Curry Soup with Roasted Chicken | D: | Small Quick Curry Soup with Roasted Chicken |
| S: | 1 Serving Postworkout Protein | S: | 1 Serving Postworkout Protein | S: | 1 Serving Postworkout Protein | S: | 1 Serving Postworkout Protein |
| B: | Small Lumberjack Scramble | B: | Small Mixed Berry Blast | B: | Small Southwest Eggs Benedict | B: | Small California Scramble |
| L: | Small Moroccan Chicken w/ Sweet Potato Fries | L: | Small Moroccan Chicken w/ Sweet Potato Fries | L: | Small Tomato and Chickpea Salad w/ New York Strip Steak | L: | Small Fat-Loss Shrimp Fajitas |
| S: | Small Upgraded Toast and Peanut Butter | S: | Small Avocado Toast | S: | Small Avocado Toast | S: | Small Berries and Cream 2.0 |
| D: | Large 3-Bean Salad w/ Grilled Garlic Parmesan Chicken | D: | Large 3-Bean Salad w/ Grilled Garlic Parmesan Chicken | D: | Large Vietnamese Salad | D: | Large Vietnamese Salad |
| S: | 1 Serving Postworkout Protein | S: | 1 Serving Postworkout Protein | S: | 1 Serving Postworkout Protein | S: | 1 Serving Postworkout Protein |

# MetaShred Meal-Planning Calendar—MetaDiet Level C; Plan 1

| | SUNDAY | MONDAY | TUESDAY |
|---|---|---|---|
| B: | Large Smooth Herbed Eggs | Small Raspberry-Pistachio Parfait | Small Crustless Bite-Size Quiche |
| L: | Small Chef Salad | Small Turkey Meatball Bowl | Small Turkey Meatball Bowl |
| S: | Small Peanut Butter Cake Batter | Small Chia Yogurt | Small Lox and Pistachios |
| D: | Small Chicken Caesar Salad | Large Sloppy Joe Bowl | Large Sloppy Joe Bowl |
| S: | 1 Serving Postworkout Protein | 1 Serving Postworkout Protein | 1 Serving Postworkout Protein |
| B: | Small Coconut-Strawberry Smoothie | Small Denver Scramble | Small Raspberry-Pistachio Parfait |
| L: | Small Grilled Chicken Salad | Large Beef Kebabs with Tzatziki Sauce | Large Beef Kebabs with Tzatziki Sauce |
| S: | Small Nuts and Beef Jerky | Small Peanut Butter Cake Batter | Small Chia Yogurt |
| D: | Large Ultimate Steak Dinner | Small Mediterranean Chicken Lettuce Wraps | Small Mediterranean Chicken Lettuce Wraps |
| S: | 1 Serving Postworkout Protein | 1 Serving Postworkout Protein | 1 Serving Postworkout Protein |

PHASE 2: FAT-LOSS ACCELERATION

| | WEDNESDAY | | THURSDAY | | FRIDAY | | SATURDAY |
|---|---|---|---|---|---|---|---|
| B: | Small All-American Breakfast | B: | Small Cheesy Scallion Scramble | B: | Small Smooth Herbed Eggs | B: | Large Death by Chocolate Smoothie |
| L: | Small Turkey Meatball Bowl | L: | Small Turkey Meatball Bowl | L: | Large Pecan-Crusted Salmon w/ Green Beans | L: | Small Herbed Tuna Salad and Avocado Bowl |
| S: | Small Nuts and Beef Jerky | S: | Small Peanut Butter Cake Batter | S: | Small Chia Yogurt | S: | Small Lox and Pistachios |
| D: | Large Mediterranean Chicken Lettuce Wraps | D: | Large Mediterranean Chicken Lettuce Wraps | D: | Small Ultimate Steak Dinner | D: | Small Curry Cauliflower w/ Seared Chicken Thighs |
| S: | 1 Serving Postworkout Protein | S: | 1 Serving Postworkout Protein | S: | 1 Serving Postworkout Protein | S: | 1 Serving Postworkout Protein |
| B: | Small All-American Breakfast | B: | Small Death by Chocolate Smoothie | B: | Small Crustless Bite-Size Quiche | B: | Small Smooth Herbed Eggs |
| L: | Small Chef Salad | L: | Small Curry Cauliflower w/ Seared Chicken Thighs | L: | Small Pecan-Crusted Salmon w/ Green Beans | L: | Small Chicken Caesar Salad |
| S: | Small Lox and Pistachios | S: | Small Nuts and Beef Jerky | S: | Small Peanut Butter Cake Batter | S: | Small Chia Yogurt |
| D: | Large Herbed Tuna Salad and Avocado Bowl | D: | Large Grilled Chicken Salad | D: | Large Sloppy Joe Bowl | D: | Large Sloppy Joe Bowl |
| S: | 1 Serving Postworkout Protein | S: | 1 Serving Postworkout Protein | S: | 1 Serving Postworkout Protein | S: | 1 Serving Postworkout Protein |

# MetaShred Meal-Planning Calendar—MetaDiet Level C; Plan 2

| | SUNDAY | | MONDAY | | TUESDAY | |
|---|---|---|---|---|---|---|
| **PHASE 1: FAT-LOSS PRIMER** | B: | Small Almond Mocha Smoothie Blast | B: | Small California Scramble | B: | Small Lumberjack Scramble |
| | L: | Small Moroccan Chicken w/ Sweet Potato Fries | L: | Small Moroccan Chicken w/ Sweet Potato Fries | L: | Small Ultimate Bibb Burger |
| | S: | Small Avocado Toast | S: | Small Berries and Cream 2.0 | S: | Small Upgraded Toast and Peanut Butter |
| | D: | Large Vietnamese Salad | D: | Large Vietnamese Salad | D: | Large Fenway Park |
| | S: | 1 Serving Postworkout Protein | S: | 1 Serving Postworkout Protein | S: | 1 Serving Postworkout Protein |
| | B: | Small Lumberjack Scramble | B: | Small Mixed Berry Blast | B: | Large Southwest Eggs Benedict |
| | L: | Small Fat-Loss Shrimp Fajitas | L: | Small Open-Faced Buffalo Burger and Salad | L: | Small Open-Faced Buffalo Burger and Salad |
| | S: | Small Upgraded Toast and Peanut Butter | S: | Small Avocado Toast | S: | Small Berries and Cream 2.0 |
| | D: | Large Spicy Green Chili | D: | Large Spicy Green Chili | D: | Small Tomato and Chickpea Salad w/ New York Strip Steak |
| | S: | 1 Serving Postworkout Protein | S: | 1 Serving Postworkout Protein | S: | 1 Serving Postworkout Protein |

| | WEDNESDAY | | THURSDAY | | FRIDAY | | SATURDAY |
|---|---|---|---|---|---|---|---|
| B: | Small Superfood Parfait | B: | Small MetaShred Smoothie | B: | Small Pumpkin Pancakes | B: | Small Pumpkin Pancakes |
| L: | Small Kung Pao Chicken | L: | Small Kung Pao Chicken | L: | Small 3-Bean Salad w/ Grilled Garlic Parmesan Chicken | L: | Small 3-Bean Salad w/ Grilled Garlic Parmesan Chicken |
| S: | Small Yogurt and Berries | S: | Small Upgraded Toast and Peanut Butter | S: | Small Yogurt and Berries | S: | Small Upgraded Toast and Peanut Butter |
| D: | Large Wedge Salad w/ Turkey Burger | D: | Large Wedge Salad w/ Turkey Burger | D: | Large Spicy Green Chili | D: | Large Spicy Green Chili |
| S: | 1 Serving Postworkout Protein | S: | 1 Serving Postworkout Protein | S: | 1 Serving Postworkout Protein | S: | 1 Serving Postworkout Protein |
| B: | Small Peanut Butter Cup Parfait | B: | Small Mixed Berry Blast | B: | Large Southwest Eggs Benedict | B: | Small Superfood Parfait |
| L: | Large Moroccan Chicken w/ Sweet Potato Fries | L: | Large Moroccan Chicken w/ Sweet Potato Fries | L: | Small Tomato and Chickpea Salad w/ New York Strip | L: | Large Ultimate Bibb Burger |
| S: | Small Berries and Cream 2.0 | S: | Small Avocado Toast | S: | Small Avocado Toast | S: | Small Berries and Cream 2.0 |
| D: | Small Fenway Park | D: | Small Vietnamese Salad | D: | Small Vietnamese Salad | D: | Small Fat-Loss Shrimp Fajitas |
| S: | 1 Serving Postworkout Protein | S: | 1 Serving Postworkout Protein | S: | 1 Serving Postworkout Protein | S: | 1 Serving Postworkout Protein |

## MetaShred Meal-Planning Calendar—MetaDiet Level C; Plan 2

| | SUNDAY | MONDAY | TUESDAY |
|---|---|---|---|
| B: | Large Smooth Herbed Eggs | Small Raspberry-Pistachio Parfait | Small Crustless Bite-Size Quiche |
| L: | Small Chef Salad | Large Mediterranean Chicken Lettuce Wraps | Large Mediterranean Chicken Lettuce Wraps |
| S: | Small Peanut Butter Cake Batter | Small Chia Yogurt | Small Lox and Pistachios |
| D: | Small Texas Chili | Small Texas Chili | Small Texas Chili |
| S: | 1 Serving Postworkout Protein | 1 Serving Postworkout Protein | 1 Serving Postworkout Protein |
| B: | Small Coconut-Strawberry Smoothie | Large Denver Scramble | Large Green Machine Smoothie |
| L: | Small Grilled Chicken Salad | Small Turkey Meatball Bowl | Small Turkey Meatball Bowl |
| S: | Small Nuts and Beef Jerky | Small Peanut Butter Cake Batter | Small Chia Yogurt |
| D: | Large Ultimate Steak Dinner | Small Mediterranean Chicken Lettuce Wraps | Small Mediterranean Chicken Lettuce Wraps |
| S: | 1 Serving Postworkout Protein | 1 Serving Postworkout Protein | 1 Serving Postworkout Protein |

**B. Breakfast  L. Lunch  D. Dinner  S. Snack**

| | WEDNESDAY | | THURSDAY | | FRIDAY | | SATURDAY |
|---|---|---|---|---|---|---|---|
| B: | Small Cheesy Scallion Scramble | B: | Large Coconut-Strawberry Smoothie | B: | Small Smooth Herbed Eggs | B: | Large Death by Chocolate Smoothie |
| L: | Large Curry Cauliflower w/ Seared Chicken Thighs | L: | Small Pecan-Crusted Salmon w/ Green Beans | L: | Small Beef Kebabs w/ Tzatziki Sauce | L: | Small Beef Kebabs w/ Tzatziki Sauce |
| S: | Small Nuts and Beef Jerky | S: | Small Peanut Butter Cake Batter | S: | Small Chia Yogurt | S: | Small Lox and Pistachios |
| D: | Small Texas Chili | D: | Small Texas Chili | D: | Large Grilled Chicken Salad | D: | Small Curry Cauliflower w/ Seared Chicken Thighs |
| S: | 1 Serving Postworkout Protein | S: | 1 Serving Postworkout Protein | S: | 1 Serving Postworkout Protein | S: | 1 Serving Postworkout Protein |
| B: | Small All-American Breakfast | B: | Small Death by Chocolate Smoothie | B: | Large Crustless Bite-Size Quiche | B: | Small Smooth Herbed Eggs |
| L: | Small Turkey Meatball Bowl | L: | Small Turkey Meatball Bowl | L: | Small Pecan-Crusted Salmon w/ Green Beans | L: | Small Chef Salad |
| S: | Small Lox and Pistachios | S: | Small Nuts and Beef Jerky | S: | Small Peanut Butter Cake Batter | S: | Small Chia Yogurt |
| D: | Large Grilled Chicken Salad | D: | Large Herbed Tuna Salad and Avocado Bowl | D: | Small Ultimate Steak Dinner | D: | Large Pecan-Crusted Salmon w/ Green Beans |
| S: | 1 Serving Postworkout Protein | S: | 1 Serving Postworkout Protein | S: | 1 Serving Postworkout Protein | S: | 1 Serving Postworkout Protein |

# MetaShred Meal-Planning Calendar—MetaDiet Level D; Plan 1

**PHASE 1: FAT-LOSS PRIMER**

|  | SUNDAY |  | MONDAY |  | TUESDAY |
|---|---|---|---|---|---|
| B: | Large Almond Mocha Smoothie Blast | B: | Large California Scramble | B: | Large Southwest Eggs Benedict |
| L: | Large Moroccan Chicken w/ Sweet Potato Fries | L: | Wedge Salad w/ Turkey Burger | L: | Large Quick Curry Soup w/ Roasted Chicken |
| S: | Large MetaShred Smoothie | S: | Large Avocado Toast | S: | Large Yogurt and Berries |
| D: | Small Fenway Park | D: | Large Tomato and Chickpea Salad w/ New York Strip Steak | D: | Small Tomato and Chickpea Salad w/ New York Strip Steak |
| S: | 1 Serving Postworkout Protein | S: | 1 Serving Postworkout Protein | S: | 1 Serving Postworkout Protein |
| B: | Large Pumpkin Pancakes | B: | Large Pumpkin Pancakes | B: | Large Pomegranate-Banana Smoothie |
| L: | Large Kung Pao Chicken | L: | Small Spicy Green Chili | L: | Small Spicy Green Chili |
| S: | Large Upgraded Toast and Peanut Butter | S: | Large Avocado Toast | S: | Large MetaShred Smoothie |
| D: | Small Wedge Salad w/ Turkey Burger | D: | Large Open-Faced Buffalo Burger and Salad | D: | Large Open-Faced Buffalo Burger and Salad |
| S: | 1 Serving Postworkout Protein | S: | 1 Serving Postworkout Protein | S: | 1 Serving Postworkout Protein |

**B. Breakfast     L. Lunch     D. Dinner     S. Snack**

| | WEDNESDAY | | THURSDAY | | FRIDAY | | SATURDAY |
|---|---|---|---|---|---|---|---|
| B: | Small Superfood Parfait | B: | Small Chocolate-Cherry Indulgence | B: | Large Pomegranate-Banana Smoothie | B: | Large Lumberjack Scramble |
| L: | Large Quick Curry Soup w/ Roasted Chicken | L: | Large Quick Curry Soup w/ Roasted Chicken | L: | Large Quick Curry Soup w/ Roasted Chicken | L: | Large Kung Pao Chicken |
| S: | Large Yogurt and Berries | S: | Large MetaShred Smoothie | S: | Large Avocado Toast | S: | Large Yogurt and Berries |
| D: | Large Vietnamese Salad | D: | Large Vietnamese Salad | D: | Small Fat-Loss Shrimp Fajitas | D: | Small Wedge Salad w/ Turkey Burger |
| S: | 1 Serving Postworkout Protein | S: | 1 Serving Postworkout Protein | S: | 1 Serving Postworkout Protein | S: | 1 Serving Postworkout Protein |
| B: | Large Almond Mocha Smoothie Blast | B: | Large California Scramble | B: | Large Southwest Eggs Benedict | B: | Small Pomegranate-Banana Smoothie |
| L: | Small Spicy Green Chili | L: | Small Spicy Green Chili | L: | Small Spicy Green Chili | L: | Large Ultimate Bibb Burger |
| S: | Large Upgraded Toast and Peanut Butter | S: | Large Berries and Cream 2.0 | S: | Large Avocado Toast | S: | Large Upgraded Toast and Peanut Butter |
| D: | Large Moroccan Chicken w/ Sweet Potato Fries | D: | Large Moroccan Chicken w/ Sweet Potato Fries | D: | Large Tomato and Chickpea Salad w/ New York Strip Steak | D: | Large Fenway Park |
| S: | 1 Serving Postworkout Protein | S: | 1 Serving Postworkout Protein | S: | 1 Serving Postworkout Protein | S: | 1 Serving Postworkout Protein |

# MetaShred Meal-Planning Calendar—MetaDiet Level D; Plan 1

| | SUNDAY | | MONDAY | | TUESDAY | |
|---|---|---|---|---|---|---|
| **PHASE 2: FAT-LOSS ACCELERATION** | B: Large All-American Breakfast | | B: Small Cheesy Scallion Scramble | | B: Small Banana-Nut Smoothie | |
| | L: Large Mediterranean Chicken Lettuce Wraps | | L: Large Mediterranean Chicken Lettuce Wraps | | L: Large Chef Salad | |
| | S: Large Nuts and Beef Jerky | | S: Large Peanut Butter Cake Batter | | S: Large Lox and Pistachios | |
| | D: Small Herbed Tuna Salad and Avocado Bowl | | D: Large Chicken Caesar Salad | | D: Large Curry Cauliflower w/ Seared Chicken Thighs | |
| | S: 1 Serving Postworkout Protein | | S: 1 Serving Postworkout Protein | | S: 1 Serving Postworkout Protein | |
| | B: Large Raspberry-Pistachio Parfait | | B: Large Smooth Herbed Eggs | | B: Large Creamy Peanut Butter Smoothie | |
| | L: Large Mediterranean Chicken Lettuce Wraps | | L: Large Mediterranean Chicken Lettuce Wraps | | L: Large Curry Cauliflower w/ Seared Chicken Thighs | |
| | S: Large Peanut Butter Cake Batter | | S: Large Chia Yogurt | | S: Large Lox and Pistachios | |
| | D: Small Turkey Meatball Bowl | | D: Small Turkey Meatball Bowl | | D: Small Turkey Meatball Bowl | |
| | S: 1 Serving Postworkout Protein | | S: 1 Serving Postworkout Protein | | S: 1 Serving Postworkout Protein | |

**B. Breakfast    L. Lunch    D. Dinner    S. Snack**

| | WEDNESDAY | | THURSDAY | | FRIDAY | | SATURDAY |
|---|---|---|---|---|---|---|---|
| B: | Small Crustless Bite-Size Quiche | B: | Small Coconut-Strawberry Smoothie | B: | Large Death by Chocolate Smoothie | B: | Small Crustless Bite-Size Quiche |
| L: | Large Beef Kebabs w/ Tzatziki Sauce | L: | Large Beef Kebabs w/ Tzatziki Sauce | L: | Small Chef Salad | L: | Large Chicken Caesar Salad |
| S: | Large Peanut Butter Cake Batter | S: | Large Peanut Butter Cake Batter | S: | Large Chia Yogurt | S: | Large Nuts and Beef Jerky |
| D: | Large Grilled Chicken Salad | D: | Large Pecan-Crusted Salmon w/ Green Beans | D: | Large Sloppy Joe Bowl | D: | Large Sloppy Joe Bowl |
| S: | 1 Serving Postworkout Protein | S: | 1 Serving Postworkout Protein | S: | 1 Serving Postworkout Protein | S: | 1 Serving Postworkout Protein |
| B: | Large All-American Breakfast | B: | Small Cheesy Scallion Scramble | B: | Large Crustless Bite-Size Quiche | B: | Small Coconut-Strawberry Smoothie |
| L: | Large Chicken Caesar Salad | L: | Large Beef Kebabs w/ Tzatziki Sauce | L: | Large Beef Kebabs w/ Tzatziki Sauce | L: | Large Grilled Chicken Salad |
| S: | Large Nuts and Beef Jerky | S: | Large Peanut Butter Cake Batter | S: | Large Chia Yogurt | S: | Large Lox and Pistachios |
| D: | Small Turkey Meatball Bowl | D: | Large Pecan-Crusted Salmon w/ Green Beans | D: | Small Herbed Tuna Salad and Avocado Bowl | D: | Large Ultimate Steak Dinner |
| S: | 1 Serving Postworkout Protein | S: | 1 Serving Postworkout Protein | S: | 1 Serving Postworkout Protein | S: | 1 Serving Postworkout Protein |

# MetaShred Meal-Planning Calendar—MetaDiet Level D; Plan 2

| | | SUNDAY | | MONDAY | | TUESDAY |
|---|---|---|---|---|---|---|
| **PHASE 1: FAT-LOSS PRIMER** | B: | Small Superfood Parfait | B: | Small Peanut Butter Cup Parfait | B: | Large Southwest Eggs Benedict |
| | L: | Large Moroccan Chicken w/ Sweet Potato Fries | L: | Large Moroccan Chicken w/ Sweet Potato Fries | L: | Large Fat-Loss Shrimp Fajitas |
| | S: | Large Upgraded Toast and Peanut Butter | S: | Large Almond Mocha Smoothie Blast | S: | Large Avocado Toast |
| | D: | Large Open-Faced Buffalo Burger and Salad | D: | Large Open-Faced Buffalo Burger and Salad | D: | Small 3-Bean Salad w/ Grilled Garlic Parmesan Chicken |
| | S: | 1 Serving Postworkout Protein | S: | 1 Serving Postworkout Protein | S: | 1 Serving Postworkout Protein |
| | B: | Large Chocolate-Cherry Indulgence | B: | Large Southwest Eggs Benedict | B: | Small Mixed Berry Blast |
| | L: | Small Kung Pao Chicken | L: | Small Spicy Green Chili | L: | Large Fenway Park |
| | S: | Large Avocado Toast | S: | Large Almond Mocha Smoothie Blast | S: | Large Upgraded Toast and Peanut Butter |
| | D: | Large Spicy Green Chili | D: | Large Open-Faced Buffalo Burger and Salad | D: | Large Open-Faced Buffalo Burger and Salad |
| | S: | 1 Serving Postworkout Protein | S: | 1 Serving Postworkout Protein | S: | 1 Serving Postworkout Protein |

| | WEDNESDAY | | THURSDAY | | FRIDAY | | SATURDAY |
|---|---|---|---|---|---|---|---|
| B: | Large Lumberjack Scramble | B: | Large Pomegranate-Banana Smoothie | B: | Large Pumpkin Pancakes | B: | Large Pumpkin Pancakes |
| L: | Large Fenway Park | L: | Small Vietnamese Salad | L: | Small Vietnamese Salad | L: | Small Tomato and Chickpea Salad w/ New York Strip Steak |
| S: | Large MetaShred Smoothie | S: | Large Avocado Toast | S: | Large Almond Mocha Smoothie Blast | S: | Large Yogurt and Berries |
| D: | Small 3-Bean Salad w/ Grilled Garlic Parmesan Chicken | D: | Large Spicy Green Chili | D: | Large Spicy Green Chili | D: | Large Spicy Green Chili |
| S: | 1 Serving Postworkout Protein | S: | 1 Serving Postworkout Protein | S: | 1 Serving Postworkout Protein | S: | 1 Serving Postworkout Protein |
| B: | Small California Scramble | B: | Small Peanut Butter Cup Parfait | B: | Large Pomegranate-Banana Smoothie | B: | Large Southwest Eggs Benedict |
| L: | Large Vietnamese Salad | L: | Large Vietnamese Salad | L: | Small Ultimate Bibb Burger | L: | Small Ultimate Bibb Burger |
| S: | Large Avocado Toast | S: | Large Almond Mocha Smoothie Blast | S: | Large Berries and Cream 2.0 | S: | Large Avocado Toast |
| D: | Large Moroccan Chicken w/ Sweet Potato Fries | D: | Large Moroccan Chicken w/ Sweet Potato Fries | D: | Large Tomato and Chickpea Salad w/ New York Strip Steak | D: | Large Fat-Loss Shrimp Fajitas |
| S: | 1 Serving Postworkout Protein | S: | 1 Serving Postworkout Protein | S: | 1 Serving Postworkout Protein | S: | 1 Serving Postworkout Protein |

# MetaShred Meal-Planning Calendar—MetaDiet Level D; Plan 2

PHASE 2: FAT-LOSS ACCELERATION

| | SUNDAY | | MONDAY | | TUESDAY |
|---|---|---|---|---|---|
| B: | Small Coconut-Strawberry Smoothie | B: | Small Cheesy Scallion Scramble | B: | Large Green Machine Smoothie |
| L: | Large Chicken Caesar Salad | L: | Large Curry Cauliflower w/ Seared Chicken Thighs | L: | Large Curry Cauliflower w/ Seared Chicken Thighs |
| S: | Large Chia Yogurt | S: | Large Lox and Pistachios | S: | Large Nuts and Beef Jerky |
| D: | Large Mediterranean Chicken Lettuce Wraps | D: | Large Mediterranean Chicken Lettuce Wraps | D: | Small Chicken Caesar Salad |
| S: | 1 Serving Postworkout Protein | S: | 1 Serving Postworkout Protein | S: | 1 Serving Postworkout Protein |
| B: | Small Creamy Peanut Butter Smoothie | B: | Large Raspberry-Pistachio Parfait | B: | Large Cheesy Scallion Scramble |
| L: | Large Texas Chili | L: | Small Chef Salad | L: | Small Beef Kebabs w/ Tzatziki Sauce |
| S: | Large Nuts and Beef Jerky | S: | Large Peanut Butter Cake Batter | S: | Large Peanut Butter Cake Batter |
| D: | Large Mediterranean Chicken Lettuce Wraps | D: | Large Ultimate Steak Dinner | D: | Large Herbed Tuna Salad and Avocado Bowl |
| S: | 1 Serving Postworkout Protein | S: | 1 Serving Postworkout Protein | S: | 1 Serving Postworkout Protein |

| | WEDNESDAY | | THURSDAY | | FRIDAY | | SATURDAY |
|---|---|---|---|---|---|---|---|
| B: | Small Crustless Bite-Size Quiche | B: | Small Death by Chocolate Smoothie | B: | Large Smooth Herbed Eggs | B: | Small Green Machine Smoothie |
| L: | Large Texas Chili | L: | Large Texas Chili | L: | Large Texas Chili | L: | Large Texas Chili |
| S: | Large Chia Yogurt | S: | Large Peanut Butter Cake Batter | S: | Large Lox and Pistachios | S: | Large Chia Yogurt |
| D: | Large Grilled Chicken Salad | D: | Large Herbed Tuna Salad and Avocado Bowl | D: | Small Grilled Chicken Salad | D: | Large Mediterranean Chicken Lettuce Wraps |
| S: | 1 Serving Postworkout Protein | S: | 1 Serving Postworkout Protein | S: | 1 Serving Postworkout Protein | S: | 1 Serving Postworkout Protein |
| B: | Large All-American Breakfast | B: | Large Denver Scramble | B: | Small Smooth Herbed Eggs | B: | Large Raspberry-Pistachio Parfait |
| L: | Small Beef Kebabs w/ Tzatziki Sauce | L: | Small Curry Cauliflower w/ Seared Chicken Thighs | L: | Large Herbed Tuna Salad and Avocado Bowl | L: | Small Ultimate Steak Dinner |
| S: | Large Nuts and Beef Jerky | S: | Large Chia Yogurt | S: | Large Lox and Pistachios | S: | Large Peanut Butter Cake Batter |
| D: | Large Chicken Caesar Salad | D: | Large Sloppy Joe Bowl | D: | Large Sloppy Joe Bowl | D: | Large Pecan-Crusted Salmon w/ Green Beans |
| S: | 1 Serving Postworkout Protein | S: | 1 Serving Postworkout Protein | S: | 1 Serving Postworkout Protein | S: | 1 Serving Postworkout Protein |

# MetaShred Meal-Planning Calendar—MetaDiet Level E; Plan 1

PHASE 1: FAT-LOSS PRIMER

| | SUNDAY | MONDAY | TUESDAY | |
|---|---|---|---|---|
| B: | Large Southwest Eggs Benedict | B: Large California Scramble | B: Large Mixed Berry Blast | |
| L: | Large Kung Pao Chicken | L: Large Kung Pao Chicken | L: Large Ultimate Bibb Burger | |
| S: | Large Almond Mocha Smoothie Blast | S: Large Berries and Cream 2.0 | S: Large Yogurt and Berries | |
| D: | Large Moroccan Chicken w/ Sweet Potato Fries | D: Large Moroccan Chicken w/ Sweet Potato Fries | D: Large Fat-Loss Shrimp Fajitas | |
| S: | 1 Serving Postworkout Protein | S: 1 Serving Postworkout Protein | S: 1 Serving Postworkout Protein | |
| B: | Large Superfood Parfait | B: Large Southwest Eggs Benedict | B: Large Peanut Butter Cup Parfait | |
| L: | Large Kung Pao Chicken | L: Large Vietnamese Salad | L: Large Vietnamese Salad | |
| S: | Large Berries and Cream 2.0 | S: Large Upgraded Toast and Peanut Butter | S: Large Almond Mocha Smoothie Blast | |
| D: | Large Ultimate Bibb Burger | D: Large Fenway Park | D: Large Fat-Loss Shrimp Fajitas | |
| S: | 1 Serving Postworkout Protein | S: 1 Serving Postworkout Protein | S: 1 Serving Postworkout Protein | |

| | WEDNESDAY | | THURSDAY | | FRIDAY | | SATURDAY |
|---|---|---|---|---|---|---|---|
| B: | Large Pumpkin Pancakes | B: | Large Pumpkin Pancakes | B: | Large Peanut Butter Cup Parfait | B: | Large Pomegranate-Banana Smoothie |
| L: | Large Open-Faced Buffalo Burger and Salad | L: | Large 3-Bean Salad w/ Grilled Garlic Parmesan Chicken | L: | Large 3-Bean Salad w/ Grilled Garlic Parmesan Chicken | L: | Large Kung Pao Chicken |
| S: | Large MetaShred Smoothie | S: | Large Upgraded Toast and Peanut Butter | S: | Large Almond Mocha Smoothie Blast | S: | Large Berries and Cream 2.0 |
| D: | Large Quick Curry Soup with Roasted Chicken | D: | Large Quick Curry Soup w/ Roasted Chicken | D: | Large Quick Curry Soup w/ Roasted Chicken | D: | Large Quick Curry Soup w/ Roasted Chicken |
| S: | 1 Serving Postworkout Protein | S: | 1 Serving Postworkout Protein | S: | 1 Serving Postworkout Protein | S: | 1 Serving Postworkout Protein |
| B: | Large California Scramble | B: | Large Chocolate-Cherry Indulgence | B: | Large California Scramble | B: | Large Lumberjack Scramble |
| L: | Large Spicy Green Chili | L: | Large Spicy Green Chili | L: | Large Spicy Green Chili | L: | Large Spicy Green Chili |
| S: | Large Yogurt and Berries | S: | Large MetaShred Smoothie | S: | Large Upgraded Toast and Peanut Butter | S: | Large Almond Mocha Smoothie Blast |
| D: | Large Tomato and Chickpea Salad w/ New York Strip Steak | D: | Large Wedge Salad w/ Turkey Burger | D: | Large Wedge Salad w/ Turkey Burger | D: | Large Ultimate Bibb Burger |
| S: | 1 Serving Postworkout Protein | S: | 1 Serving Postworkout Protein | S: | 1 Serving Postworkout Protein | S: | 1 Serving Postworkout Protein |

# MetaShred Meal-Planning Calendar—MetaDiet Level E; Plan 1

PHASE 2: FAT-LOSS ACCELERATION

|  | SUNDAY | MONDAY | TUESDAY |
|---|---|---|---|
| B: | Large All-American Breakfast | Large Crustless Bite-Size Quiche | Large Coconut-Strawberry Smoothie |
| L: | Large Chicken Caesar Salad | Large Curry Cauliflower w/ Seared Chicken Thighs | Large Herbed Tuna Salad and Avocado Bowl |
| S: | Large Lox and Pistachios | Large Lox and Pistachios | Large Nuts and Beef Jerky |
| D: | Large Curry Cauliflower w/ Seared Chicken Thighs | Large Ultimate Steak Dinner | Large Mediterranean Chicken Lettuce Wraps |
| S: | 1 Serving Postworkout Protein | 1 Serving Postworkout Protein | 1 Serving Postworkout Protein |
| B: | Large Raspberry-Pistachio Parfait | Large Smooth Herbed Eggs | Large Death by Chocolate Smoothie |
| L: | Large Turkey Meatball Bowl | Large Mediterranean Chicken Lettuce Wraps | Large Mediterranean Chicken Lettuce Wraps |
| S: | Large Nuts and Beef Jerky | Large Peanut Butter Cake Batter | Large Lox and Pistachios |
| D: | Large Chef Salad | Large Turkey Meatball Bowl | Large Ultimate Steak Dinner |
| S: | 1 Serving Postworkout Protein | 1 Serving Postworkout Protein | 1 Serving Postworkout Protein |

| | WEDNESDAY | | THURSDAY | | FRIDAY | | SATURDAY |
|---|---|---|---|---|---|---|---|
| B: | Large Green Machine Smoothie | B: | Large Denver Scramble | B: | Large All-American Breakfast | B: | Large Creamy Peanut Butter Smoothie |
| L: | Large Mediterranean Chicken Lettuce Wraps | L: | Large Beef Kebabs with Tzatziki Sauce | L: | Large Turkey Meatball Bowl | L: | Large Chef Salad |
| S: | Large Chia Yogurt | S: | Large Peanut Butter Cake Batter | S: | Large Lox and Pistachios | S: | Large Chia Yogurt |
| D: | Large Beef Kebabs w/ Tzatziki Sauce | D: | Large Grilled Chicken Salad | D: | Large Pecan-Crusted Salmon w/ Green Beans | D: | Large Turkey Meatball Bowl |
| S: | 1 Serving Postworkout Protein | S: | 1 Serving Postworkout Protein | S: | 1 Serving Postworkout Protein | S: | 1 Serving Postworkout Protein |
| B: | Large Green Machine Smoothie | B: | Large Banana-Nut Smoothie | B: | Large All-American Breakfast | B: | Large Crustless Bite-Size Quiche |
| L: | Large Sloppy Joe Bowl | L: | Large Sloppy Joe Bowl | L: | Large Curry Cauliflower w/ Seared Chicken Thighs | L: | Large Chef Salad |
| S: | Large Peanut Butter Cake Batter | S: | Large Chia Yogurt | S: | Large Peanut Butter Cake Batter | S: | Large Lox and Pistachios |
| D: | Large Chicken Caesar Salad | D: | Large Herbed Tuna Salad and Avocado Bowl | D: | Large Pecan-Crusted Salmon w/ Green Beans | D: | Large Curry Cauliflower w/ Seared Chicken Thighs |
| S: | 1 Serving Postworkout Protein | S: | 1 Serving Postworkout Protein | S: | 1 Serving Postworkout Protein | S: | 1 Serving Postworkout Protein |

# MetaShred Meal-Planning Calendar—MetaDiet Level E; Plan 2

<table>
<tr><th></th><th></th><th>SUNDAY</th><th></th><th>MONDAY</th><th></th><th>TUESDAY</th><th></th></tr>
<tr>
<td rowspan="10">PHASE 1: FAT-LOSS PRIMER</td>
<td>B:</td><td>Large Southwest Eggs Benedict</td>
<td>B:</td><td>Large Superfood Parfait</td>
<td>B:</td><td>Large Mixed Berry Blast</td>
</tr>
<tr>
<td>L:</td><td>Large Kung Pao Chicken</td>
<td>L:</td><td>Large Moroccan Chicken w/ Sweet Potato Fries</td>
<td>L:</td><td>Large Moroccan Chicken w/ Sweet Potato Fries</td>
</tr>
<tr>
<td>S:</td><td>Large Berries and Cream 2.0</td>
<td>S:</td><td>Large Upgraded Toast and Peanut Butter</td>
<td>S:</td><td>Large Avocado Toast</td>
</tr>
<tr>
<td>D:</td><td>Large Fenway Park</td>
<td>D:</td><td>Large Kung Pao Chicken</td>
<td>D:</td><td>Large Ultimate Bibb Burger</td>
</tr>
<tr>
<td>S:</td><td>1 Serving Postworkout Protein</td>
<td>S:</td><td>1 Serving Postworkout Protein</td>
<td>S:</td><td>1 Serving Postworkout Protein</td>
</tr>
<tr>
<td>B:</td><td>Large California Scramble</td>
<td>B:</td><td>Large Pomegranate-Banana Smoothie</td>
<td>B:</td><td>Large Lumberjack Scramble</td>
</tr>
<tr>
<td>L:</td><td>Large Spicy Green Chili</td>
<td>L:</td><td>Large Spicy Green Chili</td>
<td>L:</td><td>Large Vietnamese Salad</td>
</tr>
<tr>
<td>S:</td><td>Large Avocado Toast</td>
<td>S:</td><td>Large Upgraded Toast and Peanut Butter</td>
<td>S:</td><td>Large Almond Mocha Smoothie Blast</td>
</tr>
<tr>
<td>D:</td><td>Large Ultimate Bibb Burger</td>
<td>D:</td><td>Large Fenway Park</td>
<td>D:</td><td>Large Wedge Salad w/ Turkey Burger</td>
</tr>
<tr>
<td>S:</td><td>1 Serving Postworkout Protein</td>
<td>S:</td><td>1 Serving Postworkout Protein</td>
<td>S:</td><td>1 Serving Postworkout Protein</td>
</tr>
</table>

| | WEDNESDAY | | THURSDAY | | FRIDAY | | SATURDAY |
|---|---|---|---|---|---|---|---|
| B: | Large Lumberjack Scramble | B: | Large Pumpkin Pancakes | B: | Large Pumpkin Pancakes | B: | Large Peanut Butter Cup Parfait |
| L: | Large Open-Faced Buffalo Burger and Salad | L: | Large Open-Faced Buffalo Burger and Salad | L: | Large 3-Bean Salad w/ Grilled Garlic Parmesan Chicken | L: | Large Spicy Green Chili |
| S: | Large Avocado Toast | S: | Large Upgraded Toast and Peanut Butter | S: | Large Almond Mocha Smoothie Blast | S: | Large Berries and Cream 2.0 |
| D: | Large Vietnamese Salad | D: | Large Vietnamese Salad | D: | Large Spicy Green Chili | D: | Large 3-Bean Salad w/ Grilled Garlic Parmesan Chicken |
| S: | 1 Serving Postworkout Protein | S: | 1 Serving Postworkout Protein | S: | 1 Serving Postworkout Protein | S: | 1 Serving Postworkout Protein |
| B: | Large Superfood Parfait | B: | Large Chocolate-Cherry Indulgence | B: | Large Southwest Eggs Benedict | B: | Large Lumberjack Scramble |
| L: | Large Vietnamese Salad | L: | Large Moroccan Chicken w/ Sweet Potato Fries | L: | Large Moroccan Chicken w/ Sweet Potato Fries | L: | Large Ultimate Bibb Burger |
| S: | Large Berries and Cream 2.0 | S: | Large MetaShred Smoothie | S: | Large Upgraded Toast and Peanut Butter | S: | Large MetaShred Smoothie |
| D: | Large Wedge Salad w/ Turkey Burger | D: | Large Fat-Loss Shrimp Fajitas | D: | Large Tomato and Chickpea Salad w/ New York Strip Steak | D: | Large Fenway Park |
| S: | 1 Serving Postworkout Protein | S: | 1 Serving Postworkout Protein | S: | 1 Serving Postworkout Protein | S: | 1 Serving Postworkout Protein |

# MetaShred Meal-Planning Calendar—MetaDiet Level E; Plan 2

| | SUNDAY | MONDAY | TUESDAY |
|---|---|---|---|
| B: | Large Cheesy Scallion Scramble | Large Smooth Herbed Eggs | Large All-American Breakfast |
| L: | Large Chicken Caesar Salad | Large Texas Chili | Large Texas Chili |
| S: | Large Lox and Pistachios | Large Lox and Pistachios | Large Nuts and Beef Jerky |
| D: | Large Texas Chili | Large Mediterranean Chicken Lettuce Wraps | Large Mediterranean Chicken Lettuce Wraps |
| S: | 1 Serving Postworkout Protein | 1 Serving Postworkout Protein | 1 Serving Postworkout Protein |
| B: | Large Raspberry-Pistachio Parfait | Large Raspberry-Pistachio Parfait | Large Death by Chocolate Smoothie |
| L: | Large Sloppy Joe Bowl | Large Pecan-Crusted Salmon w/ Green Beans | Large Chicken Caesar Salad |
| S: | Large Chia Yogurt | Large Nuts and Beef Jerky | Large Lox and Pistachios |
| D: | Large Herbed Tuna Salad and Avocado Bowl | Large Turkey Meatball Bowl | Large Turkey Meatball Bowl |
| S: | 1 Serving Postworkout Protein | 1 Serving Postworkout Protein | 1 Serving Postworkout Protein |

**B. Breakfast     L. Lunch     D. Dinner     S. Snack**

| | WEDNESDAY | | THURSDAY | | FRIDAY | | SATURDAY |
|---|---|---|---|---|---|---|---|
| B: | Large Raspberry-Pistachio Parfait | B: | Large Green Machine Smoothie | B: | Large Crustless Bite-Size Quiche | B: | Large Denver Scramble |
| L: | Large Texas Chili | L: | Large Texas Chili | L: | Large Ultimate Steak Dinner | L: | Large Chef Salad |
| S: | Large Chia Yogurt | S: | Large Peanut Butter Cake Batter | S: | Large Lox and Pistachios | S: | Large Peanut Butter Cake Batter |
| D: | Large Curry Cauliflower w/ Seared Chicken Thighs | D: | Large Grilled Chicken Salad | D: | Large Pecan-Crusted Salmon w/ Green Beans | D: | Large Sloppy Joe Bowl |
| S: | 1 Serving Postworkout Protein | S: | 1 Serving Postworkout Protein | S: | 1 Serving Postworkout Protein | S: | 1 Serving Postworkout Protein |
| B: | Large Coconut-Strawberry Smoothie | B: | Large Green Machine Smoothie | B: | Large Banana-Nut Smoothie | B: | Large Crustless Bite-Size Quiche |
| L: | Large Chef Salad | L: | Large Beef Kebabs w/ Tzatziki Sauce | L: | Large Beef Kebabs w/ Tzatziki Sauce | L: | Large Chef Salad |
| S: | Large Peanut Butter Cake Batter | S: | Large Chia Yogurt | S: | Large Nuts and Beef Jerky | S: | Large Peanut Butter Cake Batter |
| D: | Large Turkey Meatball Bowl | D: | Large Turkey Meatball Bowl | D: | Large Curry Cauliflower w/ Seared Chicken Thighs | D: | Large Ultimate Steak Dinner |
| S: | 1 Serving Postworkout Protein | S: | 1 Serving Postworkout Protein | S: | 1 Serving Postworkout Protein | S: | 1 Serving Postworkout Protein |

# MetaShred Meal-Planning Calendar—MetaDiet Level F; Plan 1

| | SUNDAY | MONDAY | TUESDAY | |
|---|---|---|---|---|
| | **B:** Large Southwest Eggs Benedict | **B:** Large Superfood Parfait | **B:** Large Peanut Butter Cup Parfait | |
| | **L:** Large Kung Pao Chicken | **L:** Large Kung Pao Chicken | **L:** Large Fat-Loss Shrimp Fajitas | |
| | **S:** Small Fat-Loss Shrimp Fajitas | **S:** Small Mixed Berry Blast | **S:** Fenway Park | |
| **PHASE 1: FAT-LOSS PRIMER** | **D:** Large Tomato and Chickpea Salad w/ New York Strip Steak | **D:** Large Wedge Salad w/ Turkey Burger | **D:** Large Wedge Salad w/ Turkey Burger | |
| | **S:** 1 Serving Postworkout Protein | **S:** 1 Serving Postworkout Protein | **S:** 1 Serving Postworkout Protein | |
| | **B:** Large Pomegranate-Banana Smoothie | **B:** Large Mixed Berry Blast | **B:** Large Peanut Butter Cup Parfait | |
| | **L:** Large Quick Curry Soup w/ Roasted Chicken | **L:** Large Quick Curry Soup w/ Roasted Chicken | **L:** Large Quick Curry Soup w/ Roasted Chicken | |
| | **S:** Small Fat-Loss Shrimp Fajitas | **S:** Small Wedge Salad w/ Turkey Burger | **S:** Small Wedge Salad w/ Turkey Burger | |
| | **D:** Large Ultimate Bibb Burger | **D:** Large 3-Bean Salad w/ Grilled Garlic Parmesan Chicken | **D:** Large 3-Bean Salad w/ Grilled Garlic Parmesan Chicken | |
| | **S:** 1 Serving Postworkout Protein | **S:** 1 Serving Postworkout Protein | **S:** 1 Serving Postworkout Protein | |

| WEDNESDAY | THURSDAY | FRIDAY | SATURDAY |
|---|---|---|---|
| B: Large Lumberjack Scramble | B: Large California Scramble | B: Large Pumpkin Pancakes | B: Large Pumpkin Pancakes |
| L: Large Open-Faced Buffalo Burger and Salad | L: Large Open-Faced Buffalo Burger and Salad | L: Large Fenway Park | L: Large Quick Curry Soup w/ Roasted Chicken |
| S: Small Pomegranate-Banana Smoothie | S: Small Meta Shred Smoothie | S: Small Tomato and Chickpea Salad w/ New York Strip Steak | S: Small Tomato and Chickpea Salad w/ New York Strip Steak |
| D: Large Moroccan Chicken w/ Sweet Potato Fries | D: Large Moroccan Chicken w/ Sweet Potato Fries | D: Large Vietnamese Salad | D: Large Vietnamese Salad |
| S: 1 Serving Postworkout Protein | S: 1 Serving Postworkout Protein | S: 1 Serving Postworkout Protein | S: 1 Serving Postworkout Protein |
| B: Large California Scramble | B: Large Chocolate-Cherry Indulgence | B: Large Almond Mocha Smoothie Blast | B: Large MetaShred Smoothie |
| L: Large Kung Pao Chicken | L: Large Kung Pao Chicken | L: Large Tomato and Chickpea Salad w/ New York Strip Steak | L: Large Fat-Loss Shrimp Fajitas |
| S: Small Moroccan Chicken w/ Sweet Potato Fries | S: Small Moroccan Chicken w/ Sweet Potato Fries | S: Small Open-Faced Buffalo Burger and Salad | S: Small Open-Faced Buffalo Burger and Salad |
| D: Large Spicy Green Chili | D: Large Spicy Green Chili | D: Large Spicy Green Chili | D: Large Spicy Green Chili |
| S: 1 Serving Postworkout Protein | S: 1 Serving Postworkout Protein | S: 1 Serving Postworkout Protein | S: 1 Serving Postworkout Protein |

# MetaShred Meal-Planning Calendar—MetaDiet Level F; Plan 1

|  | SUNDAY | MONDAY | TUESDAY |
|---|---|---|---|
| B: | Large Denver Scramble | Large Raspberry-Pistachio Parfait | Large Smooth Herbed Eggs |
| L: | Large Texas Chili | Large Chef Salad | Large Mediterranean Chicken Lettuce Wraps |
| S: | Small Herbed Tuna Salad and Avocado Bowl | Small Curry Cauliflower w/ Seared Chicken Thighs | Small Chicken Caesar Salad |
| D: | Large Curry Cauliflower w/ Seared Chicken Thighs | Large Texas Chili | Large Texas Chili |
| S: | 1 Serving Postworkout Protein | 1 Serving Postworkout Protein | 1 Serving Postworkout Protein |
| B: | Large Death by Chocolate Smoothie | Large Crustless Bite-Size Quiche | Large Banana-Nut Smoothie |
| L: | Large Beef Kebabs w/ Tzatziki Sauce | Large Chef Salad | Large Mediterranean Chicken Lettuce Wraps |
| S: | Small Green Machine Smoothie | Small Pecan-Crusted Salmon w/ Green Beans | Small Creamy Peanut Butter Smoothie |
| D: | Large Herbed Tuna Salad and Avocado Bowl | Large Turkey Meatball Bowl | Large Turkey Meatball Bowl |
| S: | 1 Serving Postworkout Protein | 1 Serving Postworkout Protein | 1 Serving Postworkout Protein |

**B. Breakfast    L. Lunch    D. Dinner    S. Snack**

| | WEDNESDAY | | THURSDAY | | FRIDAY | | SATURDAY |
|---|---|---|---|---|---|---|---|
| B: | Large Cheesy Scallion Scramble | B: | Large Creamy Peanut Butter Smoothie | B: | Large All-American Breakfast | B: | Large Coconut Strawberry Smoothie |
| L: | Large Texas Chili | L: | Large Texas Chili | L: | Large Ultimate Steak Dinner | L: | Large Beef Kebabs w/ Tzatziki Sauce |
| S: | Small Death by Chocolate Smoothie | S: | Small Banana-Nut Smoothie | S: | Small Herbed Tuna Salad and Avocado Bowl | S: | Small Chef Salad |
| D: | Large Mediterranean Chicken Lettuce Wraps | D: | Large Chicken Caesar Salad | D: | Large Pecan-Crusted Salmon w/ Green Beans | D: | Large Grilled Chicken Salad |
| S: | 1 Serving Postworkout Protein | S: | 1 Serving Postworkout Protein | S: | 1 Serving Postworkout Protein | S: | 1 Serving Postworkout Protein |
| B: | Large Denver Scramble | B: | Large Green Machine Smoothie | B: | Large Coconut-Strawberry Smoothie | B: | Large Raspberry-Pistachio Parfait |
| L: | Large Mediterranean Chicken Lettuce Wraps | L: | Large Chicken Caesar Salad | L: | Large Pecan-Crusted Salmon w/ Green Beans | L: | Large Grilled Chicken Salad |
| S: | Small Grilled Chicken Salad | S: | Small Ultimate Steak Dinner | S: | Small Beef Kebabs w/ Tzatziki Sauce | S: | Small Beef Kebabs w/ Tzatziki Sauce |
| D: | Large Turkey Meatball Bowl | D: | Large Turkey Meatball Bowl | D: | Large Sloppy Joe Bowl | D: | Large Sloppy Joe Bowl |
| S: | 1 Serving Postworkout Protein | S: | 1 Serving Postworkout Protein | S: | 1 Serving Postworkout Protein | S: | 1 Serving Postworkout Protein |

# MetaShred Meal-Planning Calendar—MetaDiet Level F; Plan 2

| | SUNDAY | MONDAY | TUESDAY | |
|---|---|---|---|---|
| B: | Large Peanut Butter Cup Parfait | B: Large California Scramble | B: Large Lumberjack Scramble | |
| L: | Large Kung Pao Chicken | L: Large Kung Pao Chicken | L: Large Fat-Loss Shrimp Fajitas | |
| S: | Small Fat-Loss Shrimp Fajitas | S: Small Mixed Berry Blast | S: Small MetaShred Smoothie | |
| D: | Large Tomato and Chickpea Salad w/ New York Strip Steak | D: Large 3-Bean Salad w/ Grilled Garlic Parmesan Chicken | D: Large 3-Bean Salad w/ Grilled Garlic Parmesan Chicken | |
| S: | 1 Serving Postworkout Protein | S: 1 Serving Postworkout Protein | S: 1 Serving Postworkout Protein | |
| B: | Large Chocolate-Cherry Indulgence | B: Large Lumberjack Scramble | B: Large Mixed Berry Blast | |
| L: | Large Ultimate Bibb Burger | L: Large Wedge Salad w/ Turkey Burger | L: Large Wedge Salad w/ Turkey Burger | |
| S: | Small Spicy Green Chili | S: Small Spicy Green Chili | S: Small Spicy Green Chili | |
| D: | Large Fat-Loss Shrimp Fajitas | D: Large Fenway Park | D: Large Kung Pao Chicken | |
| S: | 1 Serving Postworkout Protein | S: 1 Serving Postworkout Protein | S: 1 Serving Postworkout Protein | |

**PHASE 1: FAT-LOSS PRIMER**

| | WEDNESDAY | | THURSDAY | | FRIDAY | | SATURDAY |
|---|---|---|---|---|---|---|---|
| B: | Large Almond Mocha Smoothie Blast | B: | Large Mixed Berry Blast | B: | Large Pumpkin Pancakes | B: | Large Pumpkin Pancakes |
| L: | Large Open-Faced Buffalo Burger and Salad | L: | Large Open-Faced Buffalo Burger and Salad | L: | Large Fenway Park | L: | Large Tomato and Chickpea Salad w/ New York Strip Steak |
| S: | Small Tomato and Chickpea Salad w/ New York Strip Steak | S: | Small MetaShred Smoothie | S: | Small Spicy Green Chili | S: | Large Tomato and Chickpea Salad w/ New York Strip Steak |
| D: | Large Moroccan Chicken w/ Sweet Potato Fries | D: | Large Moroccan Chicken w/ Sweet Potato Fries | D: | Large Vietnamese Salad | D: | Large Vietnamese Salad |
| S: | 1 Serving Postworkout Protein | S: | 1 Serving Postworkout Protein | S: | 1 Serving Postworkout Protein | S: | 1 Serving Postworkout Protein |
| B: | Large Southwest Eggs Benedict | B: | Large California Scramble | B: | Large Pomegranate-Banana Smoothie | B: | Large Lumberjack Scramble |
| L: | Large Moroccan Chicken w/ Sweet Potato Fries | L: | Large Moroccan Chicken w/ Sweet Potato Fries | L: | Large 3-Bean Salad w/ Grilled Garlic Parmesan Chicken | L: | Large 3-Bean Salad w/ Grilled Garlic Parmesan Chicken |
| S: | Small Superfood Parfait | S: | Small Pomegranate-Banana Smoothie | S: | Small Chocolate-Cherry Indulgence | S: | Small Peanut Butter Cup Parfait |
| D: | Large Kung Pao Chicken | D: | Large Vietnamese Salad | D: | Large Vietnamese Salad | D: | Large Ultimate Bibb Burger |
| S: | 1 Serving Postworkout Protein | S: | 1 Serving Postworkout Protein | S: | 1 Serving Postworkout Protein | S: | 1 Serving Postworkout Protein |

# MetaShred Meal-Planning Calendar—MetaDiet Level F; Plan 2

<table>
<tr><th></th><th>SUNDAY</th><th>MONDAY</th><th>TUESDAY</th><th></th></tr>
<tr>
<td rowspan="10">PHASE 2: FAT-LOSS ACCELERATION</td>
<td>B: Large Smooth Herbed Eggs</td>
<td>B: Large All-American Breakfast</td>
<td>B: Large Denver Scramble</td>
<td></td>
</tr>
<tr>
<td>L: Large Sloppy Joe Bowl</td>
<td>L: Large Sloppy Joe Bowl</td>
<td>L: Large Mediterranean Chicken Lettuce Wraps</td>
<td></td>
</tr>
<tr>
<td>S: Small Raspberry-Pistachio Parfait</td>
<td>S: Small Chef Salad</td>
<td>S: Small Chicken Caesar Salad</td>
<td></td>
</tr>
<tr>
<td>D: Large Curry Cauliflower w/ Seared Chicken Thighs</td>
<td>D: Large Curry Cauliflower w/ Seared Chicken Thighs</td>
<td>D: Large Texas Chili</td>
<td></td>
</tr>
<tr>
<td>S: 1 Serving Postworkout Protein</td>
<td>S: 1 Serving Postworkout Protein</td>
<td>S: 1 Serving Postworkout Protein</td>
<td></td>
</tr>
<tr>
<td>B: Large Raspberry-Pistachio Parfait</td>
<td>B: Large Denver Scramble</td>
<td>B: Large Banana-Nut Smoothie</td>
<td></td>
</tr>
<tr>
<td>L: Large Grilled Chicken Salad</td>
<td>L: Large Chicken Caesar Salad</td>
<td>L: Large Ultimate Steak Dinner</td>
<td></td>
</tr>
<tr>
<td>S: Small Beef Kebabs w/ Tzatziki Sauce</td>
<td>S: Small Beef Kebabs w/ Tzatziki Sauce</td>
<td>S: Small Raspberry-Pistachio Parfait</td>
<td></td>
</tr>
<tr>
<td>D: Large Turkey Meatball Bowl</td>
<td>D: Large Turkey Meatball Bowl</td>
<td>D: Large Turkey Meatball Bowl</td>
<td></td>
</tr>
<tr>
<td>S: 1 Serving Postworkout Protein</td>
<td>S: 1 Serving Postworkout Protein</td>
<td>S: 1 Serving Postworkout Protein</td>
<td></td>
</tr>
</table>

| | WEDNESDAY | | THURSDAY | | FRIDAY | | SATURDAY |
|---|---|---|---|---|---|---|---|
| B: | Large Crustless Bite-Size Quiche | B: | Large Raspberry-Pistachio Parfait | B: | Large All-American Breakfast | B: | Large Cheesy Scallion Scramble |
| L: | Large Mediterranean Chicken Lettuce Wraps | L: | Large Chicken Caesar Salad | L: | Large Texas Chili | L: | Large Texas Chili |
| S: | Small Coconut-Strawberry Smoothie | S: | Small Creamy Peanut Butter Smoothie | S: | Small Herbed Tuna Salad and Avocado Bowl | S: | Small Chef Salad |
| D: | Large Texas Chili | D: | Large Texas Chili | D: | Large Chef Salad | D: | Large Curry Cauliflower w/ Seared Chicken Thighs |
| S: | 1 Serving Postworkout Protein | S: | 1 Serving Postworkout Protein | S: | 1 Serving Postworkout Protein | S: | 1 Serving Postworkout Protein |
| B: | Large All-American Breakfast | B: | Large Smooth Herbed Eggs | B: | Large Cheesy Scallion Scramble | B: | Large Green Machine Smoothie |
| L: | Large Grilled Chicken Salad | L: | Large Mediterranean Chicken Lettuce Wraps | L: | Large Mediterranean Chicken Lettuce Wraps | L: | Large Chicken Caesar Salad |
| S: | Small Death by Chocolate Smoothie | S: | Small Green Machine Smoothie | S: | Small Beef Kebabs w/ Tzatziki Sauce | S: | Small Beef Kebabs w/ Tzatziki Sauce |
| D: | Large Turkey Meatball Bowl | D: | Large Herbed Tuna Salad and Avocado Bowl | D: | Large Pecan-Crusted Salmon w/ Green Beans | D: | Large Ultimate Steak Dinner |
| S: | 1 Serving Postworkout Protein | S: | 1 Serving Postworkout Protein | S: | 1 Serving Postworkout Protein | S: | 1 Serving Postworkout Protein |

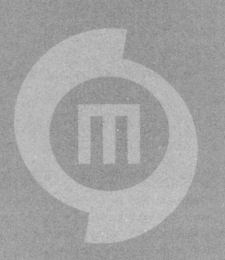

# MetaShred Diet Recipes

## Phase 1:
## Fat-Loss Primer

## Phase 2:
## Fat-Loss Accelerator

# Southwest Eggs Benedict

*Servings: 1*

Phase 1: Fat-Loss Primer

**Large Serving**

| | |
|---|---|
| 3 | eggs |
| ⅔ | cup canned black beans, rinsed |
| 1 | teaspoon ground cumin |
| 1 | teaspoon chili powder |
| 4 | slices Canadian bacon |
| 3 | slices tomato |
| 3 | tablespoons taco sauce |
| ½ | cup blueberries |

**Small Serving**

| | |
|---|---|
| 2 | eggs |
| ½ | cup canned black beans, rinsed |
| 1 | teaspoon ground cumin |
| 1 | teaspoon chili powder |
| 2 | slices Canadian bacon |
| 2 | slices tomato |
| 2 | tablespoons taco sauce |
| ½ | cup blueberries |

1. Fill a saucepan with 1" of water and bring to a slow boil. Carefully crack the eggs into the water and poach, uncovered, for about 3 minutes.

2. Meanwhile, place the beans in a microwaveable bowl and stir in the cumin and chili powder. Warm in the microwave.

3. In a nonstick skillet, heat the Canadian bacon.

4. When the eggs have finished poaching, layer on a plate as follows: tomato slice, black beans, Canadian bacon, and egg. Repeat the layering. Top with the taco sauce. Serve the blueberries on the side.

# Superfood Parfait

## Large Serving

| | |
|---|---|
| 1 | cup 2% plain Greek yogurt |
| 1 | tablespoon water |
| ¼ | cup rolled oats |
| ¾ | scoop vanilla protein powder |
| ¼ | cup pomegranate berries or ½ cup raspberries |
| ½ | cup blueberries |
| ¼ | cup cashews |

## Small Serving

| | |
|---|---|
| 1 | cup 2% plain Greek yogurt |
| 1 | tablespoon water |
| 2 | tablespoons rolled oats |
| ⅓ | scoop vanilla protein powder |
| ¼ | cup pomegranate berries or ½ cup raspberries |
| ½ | cup blueberries |
| ⅛ | cup cashews |
| 1 | tablespoon ground flaxseeds |

1. In a bowl, thoroughly mix together the yogurt, water, oats, and protein powder.

2. In a parfait glass or a serving bowl, layer as follows: yogurt mixture, berries, yogurt mixture, blueberries, yogurt mixture, and cashews. For the small serving, sprinkle the flaxseeds over the top.

# California Scramble

**Large Serving**

| | |
|---|---|
| 6 | egg whites |
| 1 | scallion, chopped |
| 2 | teaspoons olive oil |
| | Pinch of salt and black pepper |
| ½ | avocado, cubed |
| 2 | slices all-natural turkey bacon |
| 1 | grapefruit, sweetened with zero calorie sweetener of choice |
| 1 | slice sprouted grain bread, toasted |

**Small Serving**

| | |
|---|---|
| 5 | egg whites |
| 1 | scallion, chopped |
| 1 | teaspoon olive oil |
| | Pinch of salt and black pepper |
| ½ | avocado, cubed |
| 2 | slices all-natural turkey bacon |
| 1 | grapefruit, sweetened with zero calorie sweetener of choice |
| ½ | slice sprouted grain bread, toasted |

1. In a bowl, scramble the egg whites, scallion, oil, salt, and pepper. Coat a nonstick skillet with cooking spray and heat over medium heat. Add the egg mixture and stir until the whites are cooked through. Top with the avocado and remove from the pan.

2. Place the turkey bacon in the same skillet and cook completely (or, if the bacon is precooked, heat until warm).

3. Enjoy with the grapefruit and toast.

# Peanut Butter Cup Parfait

*Servings: 1*

## Large Serving

| | |
|---|---|
| 1 | cup 2% plain Greek yogurt |
| 1 | tablespoon chocolate protein powder |
| 2 | tablespoons peanut butter |
| 2 | tablespoons PB2 |
| 1 | banana, sliced |
| 1 | teaspoon chia seeds |

## Small Serving

| | |
|---|---|
| ¾ | cup 2% plain Greek yogurt |
| 2 | teaspoons unsweetened baking cocoa |
| 2 | tablespoons peanut butter |
| 2 | tablespoons PB2 |
| ½ | banana, sliced |
| 1 | teaspoon chia seeds |

1. In a bowl, thoroughly mix together the yogurt, protein powder/cocoa, and peanut butter.

2. In a separate bowl, toss together the PB2 and banana, coating the banana slices.

3. In a parfait glass or a serving bowl, layer as follows: yogurt mixture, banana slices, yogurt mixture, banana slices, yogurt mixture, and chia seeds.

# Lumberjack Scramble

*Servings: 1*

## Large Serving

| | |
|---|---|
| 3 | eggs |
| | Pinch of salt and black pepper |
| 1 | teaspoon olive oil |
| 1½ | cups frozen diced potatoes or hash browns (Simply Potatoes brand) |
| ½ | cup diced red bell peppers |
| ½ | cup diced onions |
| 3 | small precooked breakfast chicken sausage links, chopped |

## Small Serving

| | |
|---|---|
| 1 | egg |
| 3 | egg whites |
| | Pinch of salt and black pepper |
| 2 | teaspoons olive oil |
| 1 | cup frozen diced potatoes or hash browns (Simply Potatoes brand) |
| ½ | cup diced red bell peppers |
| ½ | cup diced onions |
| 2 | small precooked breakfast chicken sausage links, chopped |

1. In a bowl, scramble the eggs, salt, and black pepper.

2. Add the oil to a nonstick pan and place over medium heat. When hot, add the potatoes, bell peppers, and onions. Cook, stirring occasionally, until the potatoes are warmed through and the onions begin to turn translucent.

3. Remove from the heat and place in a bowl.

4. Coat the same pan with cooking spray and add the egg mixture and sausage. Stir until the eggs are cooked through. Add the potatoes and vegetables back to the pan and stir to combine.

# Pumpkin Pancakes

*Servings: 2*

## Large Serving

| | |
|---|---|
| 1 | egg |
| 4 | egg whites |
| 1 | cup almond meal |
| ½ | cup canned pumpkin pie mix |
| 1 | teaspoon ground cinnamon |
| 1 | teaspoon baking soda |
| | Salt |
| 1 | cup cottage cheese |
| 1 | cup blueberries |

## Small Serving

| | |
|---|---|
| 1 | egg |
| 3 | egg whites |
| ¾ | cup almond meal |
| ½ | cup canned pumpkin pie mix |
| 1 | teaspoon ground cinnamon |
| 1 | teaspoon baking soda |
| | Salt |
| 1 | cup cottage cheese |
| 1 | cup blueberries |

1. In a bowl, mix together the eggs, almond meal, pumpkin pie mix, cinnamon, baking soda, and a dash of salt.

2. Coat a nonstick pan with cooking spray and place over medium-low heat. Using a ¼ cup measuring cup, pour the batter into the pan and cook each pancake for 2 to 3 minutes. Flip and cook for another 2 to 3 minutes.

3. Serve with ½ cup cottage cheese and ½ cup blueberries on the side.

# Spicy Green Chili

### Large Serving
*(Servings: 4)*

3  tablespoons canola oil

1  medium onion, diced

3  poblano peppers, diced

1¾  pounds boneless, skinless chicken thighs

   Chili powder

   Ground cumin

   Salt and black pepper

3¼  cups salsa verde (Goya brand)

1  cup chile peppers, diced

2  cans (4 ounces each) green chiles

1¾  cups canned low-sodium chickpeas, drained

3–4 cups water, depending on thickness preference

### Small Serving
*(Servings: 5)*

3  tablespoons canola oil

1  medium onion, diced

3  poblano peppers, diced

1¾  pounds boneless, skinless chicken thighs

   Chili powder

   Ground cumin

   Salt and black pepper

3¼  cups salsa verde (Goya brand)

1  cup chile peppers, diced

2  cans (4 ounces each) green chiles

1¾  cups canned low-sodium chickpeas, drained

3–4 cups water, depending on thickness preference

1. Place a saucepan over medium heat and add the oil, onion, and poblano peppers. Cook until the onion starts to become translucent.

2. Meanwhile, dice the chicken and add it to the pan. Season as desired with the chili powder, cumin, salt, and black pepper. Stir and cook until the outsides of the chicken are cooked. You don't have to cook the chicken all the way as it will finish cooking by the time the chili is complete.

3. Add the salsa, chile peppers, green chiles, chickpeas, and water. Stir until everything is mixed thoroughly and bring to a boil for 2 minutes. Lower the temperature to a simmer and cook for 25 to 35 minutes.

# Fat-Loss Shrimp Fajitas

*Servings: 1*

## Large Serving

| | |
|---|---|
| 1 | teaspoon peanut oil |
| ½ | pound raw shrimp, shelled and deveined |
| ¼ | cup salsa |
| 1 | medium green bell pepper, sliced |
| 1 | small onion, sliced |
| ¾ | cup canned low-sodium black beans, rinsed |
| 2 | teaspoons chili powder |
| ½ | teaspoon garlic powder |
| ½ | teaspoon paprika |
| 4 | tablespoons shredded reduced-fat Colby Jack cheese |
| ½ | avocado, diced |

## Small Serving

| | |
|---|---|
| 1 | teaspoon peanut oil |
| 6 | ounces raw shrimp, shelled and deveined |
| ¼ | cup salsa |
| 1 | medium green bell pepper, sliced |
| 1 | small onion, sliced |
| ½ | cup canned low-sodium black beans, rinsed |
| 2 | teaspoons chili powder |
| ½ | teaspoon garlic powder |
| ½ | teaspoon paprika |
| 2 | tablespoons shredded reduced-fat Colby Jack cheese |
| ½ | avocado, diced |

1. Place the oil and shrimp in a nonstick pan over medium-high heat and cook until the shrimp is warmed.

2. Add the salsa, bell pepper, onion, beans, chili powder, garlic powder, and paprika. Reduce to medium heat and stir occasionally until the shrimp is cooked all the way through.

3. Remove from the heat and place in a bowl. Top with the cheese and avocado, and enjoy.

4. Note: You can make this dish even faster by purchasing precooked shrimp. Then you can simply combine all the ingredients in the pan and heat through.

# 3-Bean Salad with Grilled Garlic Parmesan Chicken  *Servings: 2*

### Large Serving

¾  pound boneless, skinless chicken thighs

2  cloves garlic, minced

1½  cups green beans

1  cup canned low-sodium kidney beans

½  cup canned low-sodium great Northern beans

4  tablespoons finely diced red onions

4  tablespoons minced parsley, divided

1  tablespoon + 2 teaspoons extra virgin olive oil

1  tablespoon apple cider vinegar

1  teaspoon Splenda

Pinch of salt

½  teaspoon black pepper

4  tablespoons Parmesan cheese

### Small Serving

9  ounces boneless, skinless chicken thighs

2  cloves garlic, minced

1½  cups green beans

⅔  cup canned low-sodium kidney beans

⅔  cup canned low-sodium great Northern beans

2  tablespoons finely diced red onions

4  tablespoons minced parsley, divided

1  tablespoon extra virgin olive oil

1  tablespoon apple cider vinegar

1  teaspoon Splenda

Pinch of salt

½  teaspoon black pepper

2  tablespoons Parmesan cheese

1. Coat a frying pan with cooking spray and place over medium heat. Add the chicken and garlic and cook until the chicken is done.

2. Meanwhile, in a large bowl, thoroughly mix the green beans, kidney beans, great Northern beans, onions, 2 tablespoons of the parsley, the oil, vinegar, Splenda, salt, and pepper. If time permits, make the 3-bean salad the night before and let it marinate in the refrigerator overnight.

3. Prior to serving, top the chicken with the cheese and the remaining 2 tablespoons parsley.

# Kung Pao Chicken

*Servings: 2*

## Large Serving

| | |
|---|---|
| 3 | teaspoons cornstarch |
| ¼ | cup low-sodium chicken broth |
| 1 | tablespoon rice wine vinegar |
| 2 | tablespoons low-sodium soy sauce (darker is better) |
| 3 | teaspoons sesame oil, divided |
| 2–3 | dried red chile peppers, chopped (this is where the heat come from, so adjust accordingly) |
| 2 | cloves garlic, minced |
| ¾ | pound chicken breasts, cubed |
| | Pinch of salt and black pepper |
| 4 | scallions, chopped |
| 5 | cups sugar snap peas |
| 1 | medium green bell pepper, cut in chunks |
| ½ | cup sliced water chestnuts |
| 2 | tablespoons minced fresh ginger |
| ¼ | cup peanuts |

## Small Serving

| | |
|---|---|
| 3 | teaspoons cornstarch |
| ¼ | cup low-sodium chicken broth |
| 1 | tablespoon rice wine vinegar |
| 2 | tablespoons low-sodium soy sauce (darker is better) |
| 3 | teaspoons sesame oil, divided |
| 2–3 | dried red chile peppers, chopped (this is where the heat come from, so adjust accordingly) |
| 2 | cloves garlic, minced |
| 9 | ounces chicken breasts, cubed |
| | Pinch of salt and black pepper |
| 4 | scallions, chopped |
| 4 | cups sugar snap peas |
| 1 | medium green bell pepper, cut in chunks |
| ⅓ | cup sliced water chestnuts |
| 2 | tablespoons minced fresh ginger |
| 2 | tablespoons peanuts |

1. In a bowl, mix together the cornstarch, broth, vinegar, soy sauce, and 1 teaspoon of the oil and set aside.

2. In a large skillet or wok, add the remaining 2 teaspoons oil and heat the chile peppers and garlic. When they are hot, add the chicken, salt, and black pepper and cook until lightly browned on all sides (but not cooked through).

3. Add the scallions, snap peas, bell pepper, water chestnuts, and ginger. Heat and stir until the snap peas begin to soften. Add the reserved cornstarch mixture and stir for 1 minute, as it thickens. Then stir in the peanuts.

# Ultimate Bibb Burger

*Servings: 1*

## Large Serving

| | |
|---|---|
| 6 | ounces 95% lean ground beef |
| 1 | teaspoon Worcestershire sauce |
| 2 | tablespoons crumbled blue cheese |
| 1–2 | tablespoons sliced jalapeño chile peppers, pickled from a jar or fresh |
| | Pinch of black pepper |
| 2 | leaves Bibb lettuce |
| 1 | tomato |
| 2 | slices red onion |
| ½ | cup cooked brown rice |
| ⅓ | cup low-sodium kidney beans, rinsed |
| 1 | teaspoon olive oil |

## Small Serving

| | |
|---|---|
| 5 | ounces 95% lean ground beef |
| 1 | teaspoon Worcestershire sauce |
| 2 | tablespoons crumbled blue cheese |
| 1–2 | tablespoons sliced jalapeño chile peppers, pickled from a jar or fresh |
| | Pinch of black pepper |
| 2 | leaves Bibb lettuce |
| 1 | tomato |
| 2 | slices red onion |
| ⅓ | cup cooked brown rice |
| ¼ | cup low-sodium kidney beans, rinsed |
| 1 | teaspoon olive oil |

1. In a bowl, mix together the ground beef, Worcestershire sauce, blue cheese, chile peppers, and black pepper and form into a patty. Broil or cook on an electric grill (such as a George Foreman Grill) to desired doneness.

2. Using the lettuce leaves as "bread" for your sandwich, add 1 slice of tomato and the red onion slices. Dice the remaining tomato and combine with the brown rice, kidney beans, and oil. Serve the rice and beans as a side with the burger.

# Tomato and Chickpea Salad
# with New York Strip Steak

*Servings: 1*

## Large Serving

| | |
|---|---|
| 12 | ounces New York strip steak |
| 1 | teaspoon salt |
| 1 | teaspoon black pepper |
| 2 | cups canned low-sodium chickpeas, rinsed |
| 3 | tomatoes, diced |
| 1 | teaspoon ground cumin |
| 2 | teaspoons lemon juice |
| 2 | tablespoons olive oil |
| 2 | tablespoons chopped fresh parsley |

## Small Serving

| | |
|---|---|
| 10 | ounces New York strip steak |
| 1 | teaspoon salt |
| 1 | teaspoon black pepper |
| 1½ | cups canned low-sodium chickpeas, rinsed |
| 3 | tomatoes, diced |
| 1 | teaspoon ground cumin |
| 2 | teaspoons lemon juice |
| 1 | tablespoon + 1 teaspoon olive oil |
| 2 | tablespoons chopped fresh parsley |

1. Let the steak warm to room temperature and trim all visible external fat. Rub both sides with the salt and pepper. Lightly coat a nonstick or stainless steel pan with fat-free cooking spray and heat over high heat. When the pan is hot, add the steak and cook for 3 minutes. Flip the steak and let it cook for 3 minutes, or until desired doneness. Remove from the heat and let it sit for 5 minutes before slicing to achieve maximum juiciness.

2. In a bowl, combine the chickpeas, tomatoes, cumin, lemon juice, oil, and parsley. Mix thoroughly.

# Vietnamese Salad

*Servings: 2*

## Large Serving

### Chicken

| | |
|---|---|
| 12 | ounces chicken breast |
| 1 | tablespoon fresh ginger |
| 1 | clove garlic |
| 1 | teaspoon sugar |
| 2 | tablespoons fish sauce |

### Sweet and Spicy Dressing

| | |
|---|---|
| 1 | tablespoon fish sauce |
| ½ | tablespoon diced or minced fresh ginger |
| 1 | teaspoon sugar |
| ¼ | cup water |
| 1 | clove garlic, diced or minced |
| 1 | red chile pepper, diced |
| 1–2 | tablespoons lime juice |
| 2 | teaspoons rice wine vinegar |
| 1 | tablespoon olive oil or grapeseed oil |

### Salad

| | |
|---|---|
| 6 | cups cabbage |
| 2 | tablespoons each fresh cilantro, peppermint, and basil (or to taste) |
| 1½ | cups grated carrots |
| ¼ | cup peanuts |

## Small Serving

### Chicken

| | |
|---|---|
| 8 | ounces chicken breast |
| ½ | tablespoon fresh ginger |
| 1 | clove garlic |
| 1 | teaspoon sugar |
| 1 | tablespoon fish sauce |

### Sweet and Spicy Dressing

| | |
|---|---|
| 2 | tablespoons fish sauce |
| ½ | tablespoon diced or minced fresh ginger |
| 2 | teaspoons sugar |
| ¼ | cup water |
| 1 | clove garlic, diced or minced |
| 1 | red chile pepper, diced |
| 2 | tablespoons lime juice |
| 2 | teaspoons rice wine vinegar |
| 1 | tablespoon olive oil or grapeseed oil |

### Salad

| | |
|---|---|
| 6 | cups cabbage |
| 2 | tablespoons each fresh cilantro, peppermint, and basil |
| 1 | cup grated carrots |
| 3 | tablespoons peanuts |

Phase 1: Fat-Loss Primer

1. To make the chicken: If your pieces of chicken are thick, pound them with a meat mallet to an even ½" thickness. In a large bowl, combine the ginger, garlic, sugar, and fish sauce. Add the chicken and let marinate for at least 20 minutes. Cook the chicken on a grill or skillet over medium-high heat until browned and cooked through, usually 3 to 4 minutes per side depending on thickness. Once cooled, shred or chop the chicken.

2. To make the sweet and spicy dressing: In a medium bowl or large jar, thoroughly combine the fish sauce, ginger, sugar, water, garlic, chile pepper, lime juice, vinegar, and oil. Allow the sugar to completely dissolve before using.

3. To make the salad: In a large bowl, combine the cabbage, herbs (to taste), and carrots. Add the chicken to the bowl and toss to combine. Add the sweet and spicy dressing to taste just before serving and top with the peanuts.

# Wedge Salad with Turkey Burger

*Servings: 2*

## Large Serving

| | |
|---|---|
| 14 | ounces 93% lean ground turkey |
| 2 | tablespoons crumbled blue cheese |
| 2 | scallions, chopped |
| 1 | teaspoon black pepper |
| ½ | large head iceberg lettuce |
| 1 | tomato, quartered or diced |
| 2 | tablespoons shelled and roasted sunflower seeds |
| 2 | tablespoons reduced-fat ranch dressing |
| ⅓ | cup canned low-sodium chickpeas, rinsed |
| 2 | 100-calorie whole wheat sandwich thins |
| | Ketchup and mustard |

## Small Serving

| | |
|---|---|
| 10 | ounces 93% lean ground turkey |
| 2 | tablespoons crumbled blue cheese |
| 2 | scallions, chopped |
| 1 | teaspoon black pepper |
| ½ | large head iceberg lettuce |
| 1 | tomato, quartered or diced |
| 2 | tablespoons shelled and roasted sunflower seeds |
| 2 | tablespoons reduced-fat ranch dressing |
| 2 | 100-calorie whole wheat sandwich thins |
| | Ketchup and mustard |

1. In a bowl, mix the turkey, blue cheese, scallions, and pepper. Form into 2 burgers and broil or cook on an electric grill (such as a George Foreman Grill) to desired doneness.

2. Meanwhile, cut the lettuce into 2 wedges. Pair each wedge with one-quarter of the tomato and sprinkle with 1 tablespoon of the sunflower seeds, 1 tablespoon of the ranch dressing, and half of the chickpeas (large serving recipe only).

3. Toast the sandwich thins, add ketchup and mustard to taste, and place the burgers inside.

# Quick Curry Soup with Roasted Chicken

**Large Serving**
*(Servings: 4)*

| | |
|---|---|
| 1⅔ | tablespoons canola or peanut oil |
| ½ | medium onion, diced |
| 2 | cloves garlic, minced |
| 2 | tablespoons minced fresh ginger |
| 2 | tablespoons curry powder |
| 2 | teaspoons salt, divided |
| 2 | teaspoons ground cumin, divided |
| 2½ | cups canned low-sodium great Northern or cannellini beans |
| 1¾ | cups crushed tomatoes |
| 1 | cup coconut milk |
| 2 | cups low-sodium chicken broth |
| 4 | boneless, skinless chicken breasts (4 ounces each) |
| 1 | can (8 ounces) crushed pineapple, in juice (not syrup) |

**Small Serving**
*(Servings: 5)*

| | |
|---|---|
| 1 | tablespoon canola or peanut oil |
| ½ | medium onion, diced |
| 2 | cloves garlic, minced |
| 2 | tablespoons minced fresh ginger |
| 2 | tablespoons curry powder |
| 2 | teaspoons salt, divided |
| 2 | teaspoons ground cumin, divided |
| 2 | cups canned low-sodium great Northern or cannellini beans |
| 1¾ | cups crushed tomatoes |
| 1 | cup coconut milk |
| 2 | cups low-sodium chicken broth |
| 5 | boneless, skinless chicken breasts (4 ounces each) |
| 4 | ounces canned crushed pineapple, in juice (not syrup) |

1. Preheat the oven to 450°F.

2. In a large saucepan over medium-high heat, add the oil, onion, garlic, and ginger and cook for 3 minutes, or until the onions start to soften. Add the curry powder, 1 teaspoon of the salt, 1 teaspoon of the cumin, the beans, tomatoes, and coconut milk and cook for 1 minute. Add the broth and bring to a boil, then reduce the heat and simmer for 15 minutes.

3. Meanwhile, rub the chicken breasts with remaining 1 teaspoon salt and cumin, cover with pineapple, and roast in the oven for 20 to 25 minutes, or until the internal temperature is 165°F.

4. Remove 3 cups of the soup and puree in a blender. Be careful not to overfill your blender as you don't want the hot liquids to splash on you. Mix the pureed portion back into soup.

5. Enjoy one chicken breast with one serving of soup.

# Moroccan Chicken with Sweet Potato Fries

*Servings: 2*

**Large Serving**

| | |
|---|---|
| 3 | medium yams/sweet potatoes (no bigger than 5" long) |
| 2 | tablespoons olive oil |
| 2 | teaspoons salt |
| 1 | teaspoon black pepper |
| 2 | teaspoons ground ginger, divided |
| 3 | teaspoons turmeric, divided |
| 2 | teaspoons ground cinnamon, divided |
| 14 | ounces boneless, skinless chicken breast |
| 8 | ounces frozen broccoli florets |
| 2 | tablespoons Parmesan grated cheese |

**Small Serving**

| | |
|---|---|
| 2 | medium yams/sweet potato (no bigger than 5" long) |
| 1⅔ | tablespoons olive oil |
| 2 | teaspoons salt |
| 1 | teaspoon black pepper |
| 2 | teaspoons ground ginger, divided |
| 3 | teaspoons turmeric, divided |
| 2 | teaspoons ground cinnamon, divided |
| 9 | ounces boneless, skinless chicken breast |
| 16 | ounces frozen broccoli florets |
| 2 | tablespoons Parmesan grated cheese |

1. Preheat the oven to 400°F.

2. Slice the yams into french fry–like strips. Place in a bowl and toss with the oil. Add the salt, pepper, 1 teaspoon of the ginger, 2 teaspoons of the turmeric, and 1 teaspoon of the cinnamon to the bowl and mix until the fries are thoroughly coated.

3. Rub the chicken with the remaining 1 teaspoon each of ginger, turmeric, and cinnamon.

4. Spread the fries on a baking sheet. Place the chicken in a baking pan. Bake both for 22 to 25 minutes, or until the chicken is cooked through.

5. Meanwhile, place the frozen broccoli in a microwaveable bowl, cover, and microwave for 5 to 6 minutes. Sprinkle the broccoli with the cheese before serving.

# Open-Faced Buffalo Burger and Salad

*Servings: 2*

## Large Serving

| | |
|---|---|
| 10 | ounces 99% fat-free ground turkey |
| 1 | egg white |
| 1 | tablespoon flaxseed meal |
| 5 | tablespoons crumbled blue cheese, divided |
| 4 | tablespoons Frank's RedHot Buffalo Wings Sauce |
| 2 | slices red onion |
| 1¼ | cups canned black beans, rinsed |
| 1 | tablespoon canola oil |
| 1 | large rib celery, diced |
| 1 | medium carrot, peeled and diced |
| 1 | cup cherry tomatoes, halved |
| 2 | teaspoons ground cumin |
| 2 | slices whole wheat bread |

## Small Serving

| | |
|---|---|
| 8 | ounces 99% fat-free ground turkey |
| 1 | egg white |
| 1 | tablespoon flaxseed meal |
| 4 | tablespoons crumbled blue cheese, divided |
| 4 | tablespoons Frank's Red Hot, divided |
| 2 | slices red onion |
| ⅔ | cup canned black beans, rinsed |
| 2 | teaspoons canola oil |
| 1 | large rib celery, diced |
| 1 | medium carrot, peeled and diced |
| 1 | cup cherry tomatoes, halved |
| 2 | teaspoons ground cumin |
| 2 | slices whole wheat bread |

1. In a bowl, combine the turkey, egg white, flaxseed meal, 2 tablespoons of the blue cheese, and 2 tablespoons of the hot sauce. Form into 2 patties and place in a large nonstick pan over medium heat. Cook 5 to 6 minutes on each side.

2. Meanwhile, dice 1 slice of the onion and place in a microwaveable bowl with the beans, oil, celery, carrot, tomatoes, cumin, and the remaining 2 tablespoons blue cheese and hot sauce. Mix together and heat in the microwave for 45 to 60 seconds, or until the beans are heated through. Divide into 2 portions.

3. Place the burger and the remaining slice of onion on 1 slice of bread. Serve with 1 portion of the salad.

# Fenway Park

## Large Serving

1   teaspoon canola oil
1   medium green or red bell pepper, sliced
1   small onion, sliced
2   lean precooked Italian chicken sausages
    Black pepper
1   slice provolone or Cheddar cheese
1   sprouted grain tortilla

## Small Serving

1   medium green or red bell pepper, sliced
1   small onion, sliced
1   lean precooked Italian chicken sausage
    Black pepper
1   slice provolone or Cheddar cheese
1   sprouted grain tortilla

1. For the large serving, heat a nonstick pan on medium-high and add the oil, bell pepper, and onion. Cook for 3 minutes, or until the onion starts to become translucent. For the small serving, heat a nonstick pan on medium and cook the bell pepper and onion for 5 to 6 minutes, to sweat the vegetables without the use of oil.

2. Slice the sausages on the diagonal and add to the pan. Cook for 1 minute. Add black pepper to taste.

3. Place the cheese on the tortilla and add the sausage mixture. Roll up and enjoy!

# Almond Mocha Smoothie Blast

*Servings: 1*

**Large Serving**

1   serving chocolate protein powder
½   medium banana, frozen
1   cup dark chocolate almond milk
¼   cup almonds
1   tablespoon ground flaxseeds
1–2 teaspoons instant coffee, 1 packet Starbucks Via, or 2 shots of Starbucks Cold Brew Coffee
½   cup nonfat plain kefir
½–1 cup water
3–4 ice cubes

**Small Serving**

1   serving chocolate protein powder
¼   medium banana, frozen
1   cup dark chocolate almond milk
⅛   cup almonds
1   tablespoon ground flaxseeds
1–2 teaspoons instant coffee, 1 packet Starbucks Via, or 2 shots of Starbucks Cold Brew Coffee
1–2 cups water
3–4 ice cubes

1. Place all the ingredients except the water and ice cubes in a blender and blend until smooth. Add the water and ice cubes depending on the thickness consistency desired.

# MetaShred Smoothie

## Large Serving

1   serving vanilla protein powder
1   cup frozen wild blueberries
1   cup nonfat plain kefir
2   tablespoons chopped walnuts
2   tablespoons ground flaxseeds
1   cup water
3–4 ice cubes

## Small Serving

¾   serving vanilla protein powder
1   cup frozen wild blueberries
1   cup nonfat plain kefir
2   tablespoons chopped walnuts
1   tablespoon ground flaxseeds
1   cup water
3–4 ice cubes

1. Place all the ingredients except the water and ice cubes in a blender and blend until smooth. Add the water and ice cubes depending on the thickness consistency desired.

# Mixed Berry Blast

*Servings: 1*

## Large Serving

1   serving vanilla protein powder
1½  cups frozen mixed berries
8   ounces full-fat plain Greek yogurt
1   tablespoon chia seeds
½   teaspoon vanilla extract
1   cup water
3–4 ice cubes

## Small Serving

¾   serving vanilla protein powder
1   cup frozen mixed berries
6   ounces full-fat plain Greek yogurt
1   tablespoon chia seeds
1   teaspoon ground flaxseeds
½   teaspoon vanilla extract
1   cup water
3–4 ice cubes

**1.** Place all the ingredients except the water and ice cubes in a blender and blend until smooth. Add the water and ice cubes depending on the thickness consistency desired.

# Chocolate-Cherry Indulgence

## Large Serving

1   serving chocolate protein powder

1½  cups frozen pitted sweet cherries (unsweetened)

1   tablespoon unsweetened cocoa

¼   cup low-fat cottage cheese

¼   cup chopped walnuts

1   cup water

3–4 ice cubes

## Small Serving

1   serving chocolate protein powder

1   cup frozen pitted sweet cherries (unsweetened)

1   tablespoon unsweetened cocoa

3   tablespoons chopped walnuts

1   cup water

3–4 ice cubes

1. Place all the ingredients except the water and ice cubes in a blender and blend until smooth. Add the water and ice cubes depending on the thickness consistency desired.

# Pomegranate-Banana Smoothie

*Servings: 1*

## Large Serving

1¼  servings vanilla protein powder
¾   cup pomegranate juice
½   frozen banana
3   tablespoons coconut milk
2   tablespoons ground flaxseeds
1   cup water
3–4 ice cubes

## Small Serving

1   serving vanilla protein powder
½   cup pomegranate juice
½   frozen banana
2   tablespoons coconut milk
2   tablespoons ground flaxseeds
1   cup water
3–4 ice cubes

1. Place all the ingredients except the water and ice cubes in a blender and blend until smooth. Add the water and ice cubes depending on the thickness consistency desired.

# Berries and Cream 2.0

*Servings: 1*

## Large Serving

½  cup nonfat plain kefir

2  tablespoons heavy cream

¼  serving vanilla protein powder

1  teaspoon Splenda (optional)

1  cup frozen mixed berries

## Small Serving

½  cup nonfat plain kefir

1  tablespoon heavy cream

1  tablespoon vanilla protein powder

1  teaspoon Splenda (optional)

1  cup frozen mixed berries

1. In a small bowl, mix together the kefir, cream, protein powder, and Splenda (if using). Pour over the berries and eat.

# Avocado Toast

**Large Serving**

1    slice sprouted grain bread
½   cup low-fat cottage cheese
½   avocado, sliced
     Salt and black pepper

**Small Serving**

1    slice sprouted grain bread
¼   cup low-fat cottage cheese
¼   avocado, sliced
     Salt and black pepper

**1.** Toast the bread. Spread with the cottage cheese and top with the avocado. Add salt and pepper to taste.

Phase 1: Fat-Loss Primer

# Yogurt and Berries

*Servings: 1*

**Large Serving**

¾  cup nonfat plain Greek yogurt
½  cup fresh or frozen blueberries
¼  cup almonds

**Small Serving**

¾  cup nonfat plain Greek yogurt
¼  cup fresh or frozen blueberries
⅛  cup almonds

**1.** Combine all the ingredients in a bowl and enjoy.

# Upgraded Toast and Peanut Butter

*Servings: 1*

**Large Serving**

1   slice sprouted grain bread
2   tablespoons peanut butter
2   tablespoons hemp seeds

**Small Serving**

1   slice sprouted grain bread
1   tablespoon peanut butter
1   tablespoon hemp seeds

**1.** Toast the bread. Spread with the peanut butter and top with the hemp seeds.

# Denver Scramble

*Servings: 1*

### Large Serving

3 eggs
½ red bell pepper, diced
1 ounce turkey bacon, cubed
1 teaspoon olive oil
¼ cup shredded Cheddar cheese
3 cups baby spinach
2 scallions, chopped

### Small Serving

2 eggs
½ red bell pepper, diced
1 ounce turkey bacon, cubed
3 tablespoons shredded Cheddar cheese
2 cups baby spinach
2 scallions, chopped
2 teaspoons olive oil

1. In a bowl, mix together the eggs, pepper, turkey bacon, and olive oil. Coat a nonstick pan with cooking spray and place over medium heat. When it's hot, add the egg mixture and scramble until the eggs begin to harden.

2. Add the cheese, spinach, and scallions and continue to scramble until the eggs are cooked through and the spinach is wilted.

Phase 2: Fat-Loss Accelerator

# All-American Breakfast

**Large Serving**

| | |
|---|---|
| 3 | eggs |
| ¼ | cup shredded Cheddar cheese |
| 2 | slices all-natural turkey bacon |
| 1 | teaspoon olive oil |
| 1 | cup fresh raspberries |
| ½ | banana, sliced |

**Small Serving**

| | |
|---|---|
| 2 | eggs |
| ¼ | cup shredded Cheddar cheese |
| 2 | slices all-natural turkey bacon |
| 2 | teaspoons olive oil |
| 1 | cup fresh raspberries |
| ¼ | banana, sliced |

1. Coat a nonstick pan with fat-free cooking spray and place over medium heat. Crack the eggs into the pan. Cook until the whites harden and the edges begin to bubble. Using a spatula, flip the eggs over one at a time. Top with the cheese and cook until the edges of the yolk harden but the middle is still liquid.

2. Meanwhile, place the turkey bacon and olive oil in a frying pan over medium-high heat and cook until done.

3. Enjoy the raspberries and banana on the side.

Phase 2: Fat-Loss Accelerator

# Raspberry-Pistachio Parfait

*Servings: 1*

## Large Serving

| | |
|---|---|
| 8 | ounces 2% plain Greek yogurt |
| ¾ | cup fresh raspberries |
| ¼ | cup pistachios, shelled |
| ¼ | cup coconut milk |
| 1 | tablespoon vanilla protein powder |

## Small Serving

| | |
|---|---|
| 8 | ounces 2% plain Greek yogurt |
| ½ | cup fresh raspberries |
| ¼ | cup pistachios, shelled |
| 2 | tablespoons coconut milk |
| 1 | tablespoon vanilla protein powder |

**1.** Mix all the ingredients together in a bowl or layer in a parfait glass, and enjoy.

Phase 2: Fat-Loss Accelerator

# Smooth Herbed Eggs

*Servings: 1*

### Large Serving

| | |
|---|---|
| 3 | eggs |
| 5 | egg whites |
| 2 | tablespoons heavy cream |
| 1 | teaspoon minced fresh rosemary |
| | Pinch of salt and black pepper |
| 1 | ounce goat cheese, crumbled |
| 1 | medium apple |

### Small Serving

| | |
|---|---|
| 3 | eggs |
| 2 | egg whites |
| 1 | tablespoon heavy cream |
| 1 | teaspoon minced fresh rosemary |
| | Pinch of salt and black pepper |
| 1 | ounce goat cheese, crumbled |
| 1 | cup blueberries |

1. In a bowl, mix together the eggs, egg whites, cream, and rosemary. Coat a nonstick pan with cooking spray and place over medium heat. When hot, add the egg mixture, salt, and pepper. Scramble until the eggs are cooked through. Mix in the goat cheese.

2. Serve with the fruit on the side.

# Crustless Bite-Size Quiche

*Servings: 1*

**Large Serving**

| | |
|---|---|
| 3 | eggs |
| 3 | egg whites |
| 2 | tablespoons heavy cream |
| 1 | tablespoon flaxseed meal |
| ¼ | cup shredded Cheddar cheese |
| 1 | cup chopped broccoli |
| ⅔ | banana |

**Small Serving**

| | |
|---|---|
| 3 | eggs |
| 1 | egg white |
| 1 | tablespoon heavy cream |
| 1 | tablespoon flaxseed meal |
| ¼ | cup shredded Cheddar cheese |
| 1 | cup chopped broccoli |
| ½ | banana |

**1.** Preheat the oven to 375°F. Coat the inside of a 6-cup muffin tin with cooking spray or, alternatively, line the muffin tin with disposable muffin cups.

**2.** In a bowl, combine the eggs, egg whites, cream, and flaxseed meal. Blend thoroughly, then mix in the cheese and broccoli. Fill each muffin cup evenly. Bake for 10 to 12 minutes, or until the tops begin to brown.

**3.** Serve the banana on the side.

# Cheesy Scallion Scramble

*Servings: 1*

## Large Serving

2   teaspoons olive oil

3   eggs

1   egg white

    Pinch of salt and black pepper

½   tomato, chopped

2   scallions, chopped

½   cup shredded Cheddar cheese

1   small apple

## Small Serving

1   teaspoon olive oil

3   eggs

    Pinch of salt and black pepper

1   tomato, chopped

2   scallions, chopped

⅓   cup shredded Cheddar cheese

½   small apple

**1.** In a bowl, mix together the oil, eggs, and egg white (large serving only). Coat a nonstick pan with cooking spray and place over medium heat. When the pan is hot, add the eggs, salt, and pepper. Scramble until the eggs are cooked through. Stir in the tomato, scallions, and cheese and cook until the cheese is melted.

**2.** Serve the apple on the side.

Phase 2: Fat-Loss Accelerator

# Texas Chili

*Servings: 5*

**Large Serving**

| | |
|---|---|
| 1¾ | pounds top round lean beef |
| ¼ | cup canola oil |
| 2 | cloves garlic |
| 1 | onion, diced |
| 2 | cans (6 ounces each) tomato paste |
| 2 | cans (4.5 ounces each) diced green chiles |
| 1 | chipotle chile pepper, diced (optional) |
| 1 | tablespoon ground cumin |
| ¼ | cup chili powder |
| 1 | teaspoon black pepper |
| ½ | teaspoon crushed red pepper |
| 3 | tablespoons unsweetened cocoa powder |
| 32 | ounces low-sodium beef broth or stock |
| 1 | cup water |
| 10 | tablespoons sour cream |

**Small Serving**

| | |
|---|---|
| 1¼ | pounds top round lean beef |
| 3 | tablespoons canola oil |
| 2 | cloves garlic |
| 1 | onion, diced |
| 2 | cans (6 ounces each) tomato paste |
| 2 | cans (4.5 ounces each) diced green chiles |
| 1 | chipotle chile pepper, diced (optional) |
| 1 | tablespoon ground cumin |
| ¼ | cup chili powder |
| 1 | teaspoon black pepper |
| ½ | teaspoon crushed red pepper |
| 2 | tablespoons unsweetened cocoa powder |
| 32 | ounces low-sodium beef broth or stock |
| 1 | cup water |
| 10 | tablespoons sour cream |

1. Trim all the visible fat off the beef and cut into cubes (no bigger than 1" x 1"). Place the beef and oil in a medium to large saucepan over medium heat and cook until the beef is browned on the edges. Remove from the pan and place in a bowl.

2. In the same saucepan, add the garlic and onion and cook until the onion softens. Add back the beef along with the tomato paste, green chiles, chile pepper (if using), cumin, chili powder, black pepper, red pepper, and cocoa powder. Stir until the spices and tomato paste are thoroughly mixed and coating the beef.

3. Add the broth or stock and water, cover, and simmer for 45 minutes. Stir and simmer, uncovered, for 45 minutes longer.

4. Top each serving with 2 tablespoons sour cream.

# Chef Salad

## Large Serving

3     cups shredded Romaine lettuce
½     cup cucumber, finely chopped
1     tomato, chopped
9     baby carrots, finely chopped
1     hard-boiled egg, quartered
3     teaspoons extra virgin olive oil
2     tablespoons red wine vinegar
1     slice Swiss cheese, cut into strips
1     slice provolone cheese, cut into strips
3     ounces roasted turkey, sliced

## Small Serving

3     cups shredded Romaine lettuce
½     cup cucumber, finely chopped
1     tomato, chopped
9     baby carrots, finely chopped
1     hard-boiled egg, quartered
3     teaspoons extra virgin olive oil
2     tablespoons red wine vinegar
½     slice Swiss cheese, cut into strips
½     slice provolone cheese, cut into strips
3     ounces roasted turkey, sliced

1. Place the lettuce on a plate and top with the cucumber, tomato, carrots, and egg. Drizzle with the oil and vinegar. Top with the cheeses and turkey.

Phase 2: Fat-Loss Accelerator

# Sloppy Joe Bowl

*Servings: 2*

### Large Serving

| | |
|---|---|
| 2 | tablespoons extra virgin olive oil |
| ½ | onion, finely diced |
| 12 | ounces 90% lean ground beef |
| ⅔ | cup tomato sauce |
| ¼ | cup ketchup |
| ½ | cup canned low-sodium black beans, rinsed |
| 2 | teaspoons ground cumin |
| 1 | teaspoon chili powder |
| 1 | teaspoon black pepper |

### Small Serving

| | |
|---|---|
| 1 | tablespoon + 1 teaspoon extra virgin olive oil |
| ½ | onion, finely diced |
| 10 | ounces 90% lean ground beef |
| ⅔ | cup tomato sauce |
| 2 | tablespoons ketchup |
| ½ | cup canned low-sodium black beans, rinsed |
| 2 | teaspoons ground cumin |
| 1 | teaspoon chili powder |
| 1 | teaspoon black pepper |

1. In a large nonstick pan, add the oil, onion, and ground beef. Cook until the beef is browned but not cooked through.

2. Stir in the tomato sauce, ketchup, beans, cumin, chili powder, and pepper and bring to a boil. Reduce the heat and simmer for 5 to 7 minutes. Serve in bowls.

# Curry Cauliflower with Seared Chicken Thighs

*Servings: 1*

## Large Serving

6   ounces boneless, skinless chicken thighs

1   tablespoon + 2 teaspoons canola oil

1   tablespoon + 1 teaspoon curry powder

½   teaspoon garlic powder

½   teaspoon ground cinnamon

3   cups cauliflower florets

½   cup low-fat plain yogurt

2   teaspoons cardamom seeds

## Small Serving

4   ounces boneless, skinless chicken thighs

1   tablespoon + 1 teaspoon canola oil

½   tablespoon + ½ teaspoon curry powder

½   teaspoon garlic powder

½   teaspoon ground cinnamon

2   cups cauliflower florets

½   cup low-fat plain yogurt

2   teaspoons cardamom seeds

1. Preheat the oven to 425°F.

2. Rub the chicken with the oil (2 teaspoons for the large serving or 1 teaspoon for the small serving), followed by the curry powder (1 teaspoon for the large serving or ½ teaspoon for the small serving), garlic powder, and cinnamon.

3. In a bowl, toss together 1 tablespoon oil, the curry powder (1 tablespoon for the large serving or ½ tablespoon for the small serving), and cauliflower.

4. Place the chicken in a baking dish and spread the cauliflower mixture out on a baking sheet. Place both in the oven and cook, stirring every 10 minutes, for 20 to 25 minutes, or until the cauliflower tips begin to brown.

5. Enjoy with a side of yogurt mixed with cardamom.

# Mediterranean Chicken Lettuce Wraps

*Servings: 2 (3 lettuce wraps per serving)*

## Large Serving

| | |
|---|---|
| 12 | ounces boneless, skinless chicken breasts |
| 4 | teaspoons extra virgin olive oil, divided |
| 1 | tablespoon dried basil |
| 3 | small tomatoes, seeds removed, chopped |
| ⅔ | cup crumbled feta cheese |
| ½ | red onion, finely diced |
| 16 | pitted kalamata olives, chopped |
| ½ | cup chopped parsley |
| 2 | cloves garlic, minced |
| 1 | teaspoon salt |
| 1 | teaspoon black pepper |
| 6 | Bibb lettuce leaves |

## Small Serving

| | |
|---|---|
| 10 | ounces boneless, skinless chicken breasts |
| 3 | teaspoons extra virgin olive oil, divided |
| 1 | tablespoon dried basil |
| 3 | small tomatoes, seeds removed, chopped |
| ½ | cup crumbled feta cheese |
| ½ | red onion, finely diced |
| 10 | pitted kalamata olives, chopped |
| ¼ | cup chopped parsley |
| 2 | cloves garlic, minced |
| 1 | teaspoon salt |
| 1 | teaspoon black pepper |
| 6 | Bibb lettuce leaves |

1. Preheat the oven to 400°F.

2. Rub the chicken with 2 teaspoons of the oil and the basil. Place in a baking dish and roast for 20 to 25 minutes, or until the internal temperature is 165°F. Remove and let cool, then cut into ½" pieces.

3. In a bowl, mix together the chicken, tomatoes, feta, onion, olives, parsley, garlic, salt, pepper, and the remaining oil. Portion onto the lettuce leaves and eat.

# Chicken Caesar Salad

*Servings: 1*

## Large Serving

6   ounces chicken tenders or sliced chicken breast

Salt and black pepper

3   cups shredded Romaine lettuce

3   tablespoons grated Parmesan cheese

3   tablespoons Caesar dressing (preferably Annie's Naturals)

1   medium pear

## Small Serving

5   ounces chicken tenders or sliced chicken breast

Salt and black pepper

3   cups shredded Romaine lettuce

3   tablespoons grated Parmesan cheese

2   tablespoons Caesar dressing (preferably Annie's Naturals)

½   medium pear

1. Season the chicken with salt and pepper. Broil or cook it on an electric grill (such as a George Foreman Grill) until the middle is cooked through and no longer pink.

2. Toss the lettuce in a bowl with the cheese and dressing. Top with the chicken.

3. Enjoy the pear for dessert.

# Beef Kebabs with Tzatziki Sauce

*Servings: 2*

## Large Serving

| | |
|---|---|
| 1 | tablespoon minced fresh thyme or 1 teaspoon dried |
| 1 | tablespoon minced fresh rosemary or 1 teaspoon dried |
| | Salt and black pepper |
| 2 | tablespoons extra virgin olive oil, divided |
| 8 | ounces top sirloin, cut into cubes |
| 1 | medium onion, cut into cubes |
| 2 | bell peppers, any color, cut into cubes |
| 2 | cups cherry tomatoes |
| 1 | cup nonfat plain Greek yogurt |
| ⅓ | cup sour cream |
| 1 | teaspoon lemon juice |
| 1 | tablespoon minced fresh oregano or 1 teaspoon dried |
| ½ | medium cucumber |
| 4 | cups baby spinach |
| ¼ | cup crumbled feta cheese |

## Small Serving

| | |
|---|---|
| 1 | tablespoon minced fresh thyme or 1 teaspoon dried |
| 1 | tablespoon minced fresh rosemary or 1 teaspoon dried |
| | Salt and black pepper |
| 2 | tablespoons extra virgin olive oil, divided |
| 6 | ounces top sirloin, cut into cubes |
| 1 | medium onion, cut into cubes |
| 2 | bell peppers, any color, cut into cubes |
| 2 | cups cherry tomatoes |
| 1 | cup nonfat plain Greek yogurt |
| ¼ | cup sour cream |
| 1 | teaspoon lemon juice |
| 1 | tablespoon minced fresh oregano or 1 teaspoon dried |
| ½ | medium cucumber |
| 2 | cups baby spinach |
| 2 | tablespoons crumbled feta cheese |

1. Preheat the broiler to high.

2. In a large bowl, stir together the thyme, rosemary, a pinch of salt and pepper, and 1 tablespoon of the oil. Add the beef, onion, bell peppers, and tomatoes and toss well.

3. Skewer the beef and vegetables on separate kebab sticks as their cooking times will vary. Also take care not to pack the food together too tightly, so they will cook evenly. Broil the kebabs for 12 to 15 minutes, rotating them halfway through. Depending on your doneness preference, you may choose to broil for a shorter time.

4. Meanwhile, in a bowl, mix the yogurt, sour cream, lemon juice, oregano, a pinch of salt and pepper, and the remaining 1 tablespoon oil.

5.  Using a cheese grater, grate the cucumber. Wrap the cucumber gratings in a paper towel and squeeze out the water/cucumber juice (don't skip this step or else the tzatziki will be watery). Add the drained cucumbers to the yogurt mixture.

6.  Serve the kebabs over a bed of spinach. Top with feta cheese, serve tzatziki sauce on the side, and enjoy.

# Ultimate Steak Dinner

*Servings: 1*

## Large Serving

| | |
|---|---|
| 1 | tablespoon + 1 teaspoon extra virgin olive oil |
| ½ | medium onion, halved and thinly sliced |
| 1½ | cups mushrooms, sliced |
| 2 | tablespoons crumbled blue cheese |
| 1 | tablespoon soy sauce |
| 6 | ounces top sirloin |
| 2 | teaspoons garlic powder |
| 2 | teaspoons salt |
| 2 | teaspoons black pepper |

## Small Serving

| | |
|---|---|
| 1 | tablespoon extra virgin olive oil |
| ½ | medium onion, halved and thinly sliced |
| 1 | cup mushrooms, sliced |
| 1 | tablespoon crumbled blue cheese |
| 1 | tablespoon soy sauce |
| 5 | ounces top sirloin |
| 2 | teaspoons garlic powder |
| 2 | teaspoons salt |
| 2 | teaspoons black pepper |

1. In a nonstick pan over medium heat, place the oil, onion, mushrooms, blue cheese, and soy sauce. Cook, stirring occasionally, for 20 minutes, or until the onions are translucent/brown and the mushrooms soften and become a deeper brown (the volume of the onions and mushrooms will greatly reduce as they cook).

2. Meanwhile, rub the steak on both sides with the garlic powder, salt, and pepper. Heat a frying pan over medium-high heat. When the pan is hot, add the steak and cook for 4 minutes. Flip the steak and cook for 3 minutes. Depending on the thickness of the steak, this cooking method will yield a medium doneness. Remove the steak from the pan and let it sit for at least 5 minutes before cutting and eating.

3. Finish the dish by pouring the onion-mushroom mixture over the steak.

# Turkey Meatball Bowl

*Servings: 4*

## Large Serving

| | |
|---|---|
| 1 | pound ground turkey |
| ¼ | cup flaxseed meal |
| 2 | tablespoons tomato paste |
| ¼ | medium onion, finely diced |
| 3 | cloves garlic, minced |
| 2 | eggs |
| 3 | tablespoons grated Parmesan cheese |
| 1 | tablespoon dried oregano |
| 1 | cup dried parsley |
| 3 | tablespoons extra virgin olive oil |
| 8 | ounces mozzarella cheese, cut into small cubes |
| 12 | plum tomatoes, chopped |
| ¼ | cup fresh basil |
| 1 | tablespoon balsamic vinegar |
| | Pinch of salt and black pepper |

## Small Serving

| | |
|---|---|
| ¾ | pound ground turkey |
| 2 | tablespoons flaxseed meal |
| 2 | tablespoons tomato paste |
| ¼ | medium onion, finely diced |
| 3 | cloves garlic, minced |
| 1 | egg |
| 3 | tablespoons grated Parmesan cheese |
| 1 | tablespoon dried oregano |
| 1 | cup dried parsley |
| 2 | tablespoons + 2 teaspoons extra virgin olive oil |
| 8 | ounces mozzarella cheese, cut into small cubes |
| 10 | plum tomatoes, chopped |
| ¼ | cup fresh basil |
| 1 | tablespoon balsamic vinegar |
| | Pinch of salt and black pepper |

1. Preheat the oven to 400°F.

2. In a bowl, combine the turkey, flaxseed meal, tomato paste, onion, garlic, egg(s), Parmesan, oregano, parsley, and 2 tablespoons of the oil. Thoroughly mix the ingredients. Roll the mixture into 12 meatballs.

3. Place on a baking pan and bake for 17 minutes, or until the juices are clear or the internal temperature is 160°F.

4. Meanwhile, in a bowl combine the mozzarella, tomatoes, basil, vinegar, salt, pepper, and the remaining oil. Mix thoroughly to ensure that the oil and vinegar are completely coating the tomatoes and cheese.

5. Serve the meatballs with the tomato-mozzarella salad.

# Pecan-Crusted Salmon with Green Beans

*Servings: 1*

## Large Serving

| | |
|---|---|
| 6 | ounces salmon fillet |
| 2 | tablespoons ground or finely chopped pecans |
| 1 | tablespoon Dijon mustard |
| 1 | teaspoon extra virgin olive oil |
| 2 | cups green beans |
| 1 | teaspoon paprika |
| | Salt and black pepper |

## Small Serving

| | |
|---|---|
| 5 | ounces salmon fillet |
| 1 | tablespoon ground or finely chopped pecans |
| 1 | tablespoon Dijon mustard |
| 1 | teaspoon extra virgin olive oil |
| 1½ | cups green beans |
| 1 | teaspoon paprika |
| | Salt and black pepper |

1. Preheat the oven to 375°F.

2. Place the salmon in a shallow baking dish and add 2 tablespoons water to the dish. In a small bowl, mix together the pecans and mustard and spread over the salmon. Bake for 12 to 15 minutes.

3. Meanwhile, place the oil and green beans in a nonstick frying pan over medium heat. Season with paprika, salt, and pepper and cook for 3 to 4 minutes (or longer if you are using frozen beans).

# Grilled Chicken Salad

*Servings: 1*

## Large Serving

| | |
|---|---|
| 4 | ounces boneless, skinless chicken breast |
| | Salt and black pepper |
| 2 | scallions |
| 2 | tablespoons sliced or slivered almonds |
| 4 | cups baby spinach |
| ½ | cucumber, chopped |
| 1 | tomato, chopped |
| 1 | ounce sharp Cheddar cheese, cut into small cubes |
| 1 | tablespoon extra virgin olive oil |
| 1 | tablespoon balsamic or red wine vinegar |

## Small Serving

| | |
|---|---|
| 3 | ounces boneless, skinless chicken breast |
| | Salt and black pepper |
| 1 | scallion |
| 1 | tablespoon sliced or slivered almonds |
| 4 | cups baby spinach |
| ½ | cucumber, chopped |
| 1 | tomato, chopped |
| 1 | ounce sharp Cheddar cheese, cut into small cubes |
| 2 | teaspoons extra virgin olive oil |
| 1 | tablespoon balsamic or red wine vinegar |

1. Season the chicken with salt and pepper. Place on an outdoor or electric grill (such as a George Foreman Grill) and cook until the internal temperature is 165°F. Depending on the thickness of the chicken, the cooking time could range between 5 and 10 minutes. Once the chicken is cooked, remove and let sit for 3 to 5 minutes before slicing (this ensures maximum juiciness).

2. Meanwhile, in a bowl, combine the scallion(s), almonds, spinach, cucumber, tomato, cheese, oil, and vinegar.

3. Serve the chicken on top of the salad.

# Herbed Tuna Salad and Avocado Bowl

*Servings: 1*

**Large Serving**

| | |
|---|---|
| 5 | ounces chunk white, water-packed canned tuna |
| 2 | tablespoons light canola mayonnaise |
| 1 | rib celery, chopped |
| 1 | teaspoon fresh dill |
| ½ | teaspoon black pepper |
| | Pinch of salt |
| 2 | cups spinach |
| ¼ | cup canned low-sodium chickpeas |
| ½ | cup chopped cucumbers |
| 1 | avocado, peeled and chopped |
| 5 | cherry tomatoes |
| 1 | tablespoon red wine vinegar |

**Small Serving**

| | |
|---|---|
| 4 | ounces chunk white, water-packed canned tuna |
| 3 | tablespoons light canola mayonnaise |
| 1 | rib celery, chopped |
| 1 | teaspoon fresh dill |
| ½ | teaspoon black pepper |
| | Pinch of salt |
| 2 | cups spinach |
| ¼ | cup canned low-sodium chickpeas |
| ½ | cup chopped cucumbers |
| ½ | avocado, peeled and chopped |
| 5 | cherry tomatoes |
| 1 | tablespoon red wine vinegar |

1. In a bowl, combine the tuna, mayo, celery, dill, pepper, and salt.

2. In a separate bowl, toss the spinach, chickpeas, cucumbers, avocado, tomatoes, and vinegar. Top with the tuna salad.

# Green Machine Smoothie

*Servings: 1*

**Large Serving**

| | |
|---|---|
| 1 | serving vanilla protein powder |
| 1 | cup kale |
| ¼ | cup walnuts |
| ½ | apple, peeled |
| ½ | avocado, peeled, seeded |
| 1½ | cups water |
| 3 | ice cubes |

**Small Serving**

| | |
|---|---|
| ¾ | serving vanilla protein powder |
| 1 | cup kale |
| 3 | tablespoons walnuts |
| ¼ | apple, peeled |
| ½ | avocado, peeled, seeded |
| 1½ | cups water |
| 3 | ice cubes |

1. Place all the ingredients except the water and ice cubes in a blender and blend until smooth. Add the water and ice cubes depending on the thickness consistency desired.

# Banana-Nut Smoothie

*Servings: 1*

## Large Serving

| | |
|---|---|
| 1 | serving vanilla protein powder |
| 3 | tablespoons walnuts |
| ¼ | cup almonds |
| ⅔ | banana |
| 2 | cups water |
| 3–4 | ice cubes |

## Small Serving

| | |
|---|---|
| ¾ | serving vanilla protein powder |
| 3 | tablespoons walnuts |
| ⅛ | cup almonds |
| ½ | banana |
| 2 | cups water |
| 3–4 | ice cubes |

1. Place all the ingredients except the water and ice cubes in a blender and blend until smooth. Add the water and ice cubes depending on the thickness consistency desired.

# Death by Chocolate Smoothie

*Servings: 1*

## Large Serving

| | |
|---|---|
| 1 | serving chocolate protein powder |
| 3 | tablespoons walnuts |
| ¼ | cup almonds |
| 2 | tablespoons cocoa powder, unsweetened |
| 2 | tablespoons cacao nibs |
| 2 | cups water |
| 4 | ice cubes |

## Small Serving

| | |
|---|---|
| ¾ | serving chocolate protein powder |
| 3 | tablespoons walnuts |
| ⅛ | cup almonds |
| 2 | tablespoons cocoa powder, unsweetened |
| 2 | tablespoons cacao nibs |
| 2 | cups water |
| 4 | ice cubes |

1. Place all the ingredients except the water and ice cubes in a blender and blend until smooth. Add the water and ice cubes depending on the thickness consistency desired.

# Creamy Peanut Butter Smoothie

*Servings: 1*

## Large Serving

⅓   serving vanilla protein powder

½   cup full-fat cottage cheese

2   tablespoons natural peanut butter

3   tablespoons PB2 (powdered peanut butter)

1   tablespoon chia seeds

1   tablespoon flaxseed meal

1½   cups water

3   ice cubes

## Small Serving

⅓   serving vanilla protein powder

¼   cup full-fat cottage cheese

2   tablespoons natural peanut butter

3   tablespoons PB2 (powdered peanut butter)

1   tablespoon chia seeds

1½   cups water

3   ice cubes

1. Place all the ingredients except the water and ice cubes in a blender and blend until smooth. Add the water and ice cubes depending on the thickness consistency desired.

# Coconut-Strawberry Smoothie

*Servings: 1*

**Large Serving**

| | |
|---|---|
| 1 | serving vanilla protein powder |
| 1 | cup strawberries |
| 3 | tablespoons walnuts |
| 1 | tablespoon flaxseed meal |
| 2 | cups So Delicious coconut milk, unsweetened |
| ¼ | cup light coconut milk |
| 4 | ice cubes |

**Small Serving**

| | |
|---|---|
| ¾ | serving vanilla protein powder |
| 1 | cup strawberries |
| 2 | tablespoons walnuts |
| 1 | tablespoon flaxseed meal |
| 1 | cup So Delicious coconut milk, unsweetened |
| ⅓ | cup light coconut milk |
| 4 | ice cubes |

1. Place all the ingredients except the ice cubes in a blender and blend until smooth. Add the ice cubes depending on thickness consistency desired.

# Peanut Butter Cake Batter

*Servings: 1*

### Large Serving

½  serving vanilla protein powder

2  tablespoons powdered peanut butter

1  tablespoon peanut butter

1  tablespoon ground flaxseeds

2–4 tablespoons water

### Small Serving

⅓  serving vanilla protein powder

1  tablespoon powdered peanut butter

1  tablespoon peanut butter

2  teaspoons ground flaxseeds

2–4 tablespoons water

**1.** In a small bowl, mix the protein powder, powdered peanut butter, peanut butter, and flaxseeds with a fork. Once the peanut butter is thoroughly mixed, begin adding water, 1 tablespoon at a time, until the consistency is that of cake batter.

# Lox and Pistachios

*Servings: 1*

### Large Serving

3  ounces lox (smoked salmon)

⅓  cup shelled pistachios

### Small Serving

1  0.5 ounce lox (smoked salmon)

¼  cup shelled pistachios

**1.** Eat!

# Nuts and Beef Jerky

*Servings: 1*

## Large Serving

¼   cup almonds
1    0.5 ounce peppered beef jerky

**1.** Eat!

# Chia Yogurt

*Servings: 1*

## Large Serving

1    cup full-fat plain Greek yogurt
1    tablespoon chia seeds

**1.** Combine and enjoy.

## Small Serving

⅛   cup almonds
1    ounce peppered beef jerky

## Small Serving

½   cup full-fat plain Greek yogurt
1    tablespoon chia seeds

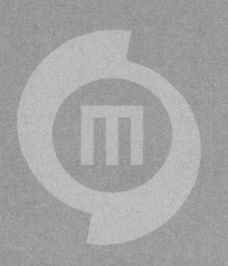

## CHAPTER 9

# Eating on the Go

I grew up in rural Vermont, where there weren't a lot of places to eat besides the deli counter at the local general store that was 3 miles away. When I was a kid, eating out at a restaurant was such a big deal. I still vividly remember one evening in which my father and I traveled more than 60 miles to Burlington to watch my older cousin play basketball, and we ate dinner at Pizza Hut before the game. I remember everything about that meal. You know eating out is rare when you have a detailed 22-year-old memory of a Super Supreme Deep Dish Pizza and a Sprite.

Whether it was an out-of-the-ordinary experience, like my childhood trip to Pizza Hut, or celebrating a special occasion or big milestone, eating out used to be an event. So, of course, you would get an appetizer, entrée, and dessert: You were celebrating!

Trouble is, times have changed. So much so that many people rarely prepare their own meals. In fact, so many people are eating meals away from home that it's almost the norm. At one point, when my client load was full of people living in New York City, I only had three clients who actually cooked; everyone else either ate out or ordered in.

Unfortunately, even though eating out is a part of everyday life for many people, the experience is still treated more like a special occasion. That leads to overindulgent meals that can easily have more than 1,000 calories. Your charge: Change your mind-set from this point forward.

# The Dining Out Deception

If you eat out a lot, you need to be wary of the dining-out deception. Don't trick yourself into thinking that because you're eating at a restaurant, you're celebrating. If you eat dinner out every night, it isn't a special event that warrants appetizer, entrée, and dessert. It's just dinner.

The hard truth is that if you eat out a lot on the MetaShred Diet, it will probably hinder your progress. The calorie and macronutrient variability of eating out is massive. You get much greater precision with your nutrition when you cook for yourself.

Eating out often may just be part of your life that you can't or don't want to change. That's fine. My good friend and celebrity trainer Joe Dowdell always tells his clients, "You just have to do the best with what you have." In this chapter, I'm going to give you the tools to do just that.

# The What-the-Hell? Effect

In the field of eating psychology, there's a concept called counter-regulatory eating. This is when someone eats a food or amount of food that they view as "bad" or "forbidden." The logical next step after overeating would be to eat less at your next meal. That way, you can account for the food that you've overconsumed, and the single deviation from your diet isn't as impactful. But you have to love the illogical beings that humans are, because with counter-regulatory eating, the initial dive into indulgence drives the person to overeat more, not less. This phenomenon is enhanced during periods of high stress.

Think of it this way: You're crushing it on your MetaShred Diet. Then, you see pizza. And not just any pizza, but your favorite pizza. You have one slice. You think to yourself, "Agh! Why did I eat that slice?" Then you say, "What the hell? I'm already off my diet, I might as well have five more slices."

This is counter-regulatory eating, or as it is more commonly called, the what-the-hell? effect.

When you're eating out, you need to avoid the what-the-hell? effect. There's a big difference between eating one slice of pizza and a whole pizza. There's a big difference between making the best choice from a bad menu versus doubling down on a triple cheeseburger with gravy fries. If you can follow Dowdell's advice and do the best with what you have, you'll be ahead of the game when you're eating out.

## Your Restaurant Survival Guide

When you go out to eat, remember that the top priority on the chef's list that night isn't making you a calorie-controlled meal. I once consulted with a new restaurant that wanted to make a fresh, local, healthy menu. I quickly learned that there were a handful of other restaurants in the area doing the same concept. However, their idea of healthy had nothing to do with controlling portions and calories while powering with protein.

No, it was all about the buzzwords that could be tagged onto the food: local, fresh, organic, farmers' market, free-range, antibiotic-free. So, yes, they may have purchased locally grown organic potatoes at the farmers' market and then cooked them in free-range duck fat. But guess what? They're still french fries.

Cooking *healthy* isn't going to be in the top three priorities on the chef's list. (The top three are probably taste/flavor, food cost, and profit.) When you go out to eat, know that the chef's version of healthy and the MetaShred Diet version of healthy probably don't meet up. This just means that you need to be extra-vigilant with how you order and how your food is prepared. Interestingly, one survey showed that 93 percent of chefs think that they could reduce the calorie content of their meals by 10 to 20 percent without customers ever knowing.[1] But they aren't doing this!

## Customize Your Order

The number one rule for eating out is to speak up for yourself when ordering. You're paying for the food, so ask for it how you like it. I've never heard of any restaurant refusing to omit the rice and add more vegetables to a dish. Don't want to be tempted by the bread basket? Just ask them not to bring it, or have them take it away if they do bring it.

## Decode the Menu

Very often, how a food is described on a menu will give you a lot of information about how it is prepared and, thus, how calorically dense the meal will be.

Avoid foods with these words in their descriptions:

- Au gratin
- Battered
- Béarnaise
- Bisque
- Breaded
- Crisp
- Fried
- Parmesan
- Scalloped

Meals described in this fashion are going to be higher in calories and prepared using more fat. When you see them on the menu, look for other options.

Pick foods described as:

- Au jus
- Baked
- Braised
- Broiled
- Grilled
- Lean
- Poached
- Steamed

## Beware of Salads

Don't automatically assume that because you're ordering a salad, it will be a calorie-conscious, portion-controlled meal. A "Farmers' Market Salad with Chicken" sounds really healthy and like an optimal meal for you on the MetaShred Diet. But, if it's drenched in dressing, full of breaded and fried pieces of chicken, and topped with sugar-coated pecans and a whole tub of goat cheese, it isn't the meal for you.

Always ask for the salad dressing on the side, and be wary of having too many fat-containing items on your salad. Fat is great and satiating, but getting avocado, almonds, and feta cheese on your salad—plus the salad dressing—will send the fat and calorie content of your meal through the roof! Pick one, plus the dressing.

## Monitor Your Portions

Remember that the portions you're served are not necessarily the portions that are appropriate for you. You aren't 10, and you're not at your grandmother's kitchen table, so you don't need to be a member of the clean-plate club.

Almost no chef has any real training in nutrition. This is illustrated by the fact that in one study, 76 percent of chefs thought that the portions of pasta and steak they were serving were regular, but they were actually two to four times what would be considered a normal serving.[2]

Generally, choose a main dish that's based around protein—beef, chicken, pork, or fish. Opt for protein that's the size of an iPhone. If you're ordering a steak, this generally means that you will need to save one-half to one-third of the portion you are served for later. (You want about 5 ounces.) That's because beef is the only protein that's overserved when it comes to portion size. Trim the external fat from your meats whenever possible, as chefs are always heavy handed with oils when cooking. So you're getting plenty of fat independent of the external fat on your meat.

Chicken is usually served in this smartphone portion size, but fish is generally underserved. Be aware of this, and don't be afraid to ask about the portion size. If it's only 3 or 4 ounces, ask for more—they'll give it to you for an upcharge.

## Indulge in Green Vegetables

When eating out, vegetables are your friends. The research on eating behavior by Barbara J. Rolls, PhD, at Pennsylvania State University is pretty clear and consistent: The more vegetables you eat—preferably green leafy ones—the less calories you're going to eat.

When eating out, always look to pile on the vegetables. This means starting off your meal with a salad. Not a salad with bacon, cheese, eggs, avocados, walnuts, and salad dressing. A simple "house" salad with lots of greens. Dr. Rolls's research shows that having a salad before a meal can decrease the total number of calories that you eat by 10 to 12 percent.[3] If you aren't big on salads, her research shows similar results with broth-based vegetable soups.

Eating more vegetables isn't a free pass to eat as much as you want. As Dr. Rolls once counseled me, your satiety signals are always there. Eating more vegetables helps strengthen these signals, but in the end, it's up to you to listen to them.

So eat more vegetables when you eat out, and use them to displace starches—which restaurants serve copious amounts of—but always listen to your body.

## Do Your Research

Many restaurants have their menus online, and more and more are providing nutrition facts for meals and individual items. Some even have "meal-builders," where you can construct a meal and it will tell how many calories it has. Panera Bread has an app for your phone that will calculate the nutrition facts for your meal and then order the food for you.

Please take the nutrition facts provided by restaurants with a grain of salt, though. I'm sure that the spoonful of guacamole that was slapped onto your riceless burrito bowl wasn't weighed or measured per the nutrition specs on the Web site.

When you're eating out, use these targets for the different phases and meal sizes on the MetaShred Diet.

## Phase 1

### Large Breakfast

- Protein: 40 grams
- Carbohydrate: 55 to 60 grams
- Fat: 20 grams

### Large Lunch/Dinner

- Protein: 45 to 50 grams
- Carbohydrate: 45 to 50 grams
- Fat: 20 grams

### Small Breakfast/Lunch/Dinner

- Protein: 35 to 39 grams
- Carbohydrate: 35 to 39 grams
- Fat: 16 to 17 grams

## Phase 2

### Large Breakfast

- Protein: 40 grams
- Carbohydrate: 30 grams
- Fat: 30 to 35 grams

### Large Lunch/Dinner

- Protein: 40 to 45 grams
- Carbohydrate: 28 to 30 grams
- Fat: 30 to 33 grams

### Small Breakfast/Lunch/Dinner

- Protein: 32 to 36 grams
- Carbohydrate: 21 to 24 grams
- Fat: 25 grams

For any of these, I recommend aiming on the low side of the numbers, particularly for fat. The idea is to get close, without going over. If you're not sure where to start, there's an app called Tell Me Food. You can enter the macronutrient parameters from pages 214 and 215, and the app will search places in your area to find items that are close to your goals.

Even if you aren't able to source a meal's nutrition facts ahead of time, you can try to estimate the portion sizes that you're served, and then enter them into a calorie-counting app like MyFitnessPal. Again, this isn't perfect, but it's doing the best with what you have to work with.

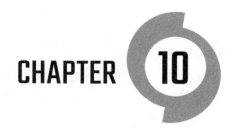

CHAPTER 10

# Day 29: Now What?

Early in my career, when I was consulting with people about their diets, I had a pivotal conversation. It made me realize how important it is for me to help clients develop the right mind-set for lifelong leanness, versus just helping them manage their diets so they could lose weight. I had been working with this client for a couple of months, and she had made great progress with her fat loss. During one of our biweekly check-ins, she was talking about how happy she was with her progress, but that she was looking forward to reaching her goals so she could go back to eating "normal" again.

Flag on the play! Specifically, the part about "back to eating *normal* again." We then went on to have a great conversation about how there was no going "back to *normal* eating" and that, in fact, the work we had been doing together for the past several months was laying the foundation for a new "*normal.*"

There's some interesting data to support the importance of this outlook shift. In Greece, there is a weight-loss registry containing a curated voluntary database of people who have lost at least 10 percent of their body weight and maintained that weight loss for at least 1 year. The United States has a similar database called the National Weight Control Registry. Countries curate databases of these people, since they are the unicorns of weight loss. Researchers then study their habits and behaviors to see what makes them successful at weight maintenance—something that is elusive to so many millions of people.

Researchers from Harokopio University in Athens have completed multiple in-depth analyses of the differences between weight-maintainers versus regainers. One of the most poignant that I have read comes from the conclusion of their 2013 analysis published in *Clinical Obesity*.[1] They concluded that: "Maintainers continuously applied specific strategies to maintain their weight. . . . Regainers considered the behaviours leading to weight loss different from their normal lifestyles, and resumed their old habits when the diet was over."

This is "back to normal" versus "new normal" in spades.

The other finding that stuck out to me was that weight-maintainers and regainers deal with the same issues—emotional eating, lack of time to exercise, wavering motivation. However, the weight-maintainers discovered ways to compensate for their emotional eating. They might eat a little less at the next meal, found time to exercise consistently, and followed through on their portion-controlled plan despite lack of motivation. It reminds me of businessman and self-improvement author Brian Tracy who says that successful people and unsuccessful people don't like to do the same things, but successful people do them anyway.

The choice is up to you.

When you go on the MetaShred Diet, your body changes and you lose fat because it is different than what you were doing previously. If you go back to what you had been doing, your body will revert back to its old self. This is a hard truth about dieting and nutrition that many people fail to grasp. There's a direct correlation between your eating and physical activity behaviors and your weight. When you lose weight, that relationship doesn't go away, it is in fact stronger than ever. Your metabolism is arguably more fragile right after you finish any diet, as there are master regulating systems that are trying to push your body back to its old bodyweight set point.

Herein lies the problem with most diets: They are proposed as short-term changes for a lifelong endeavor. So here's what I'm asking from you.

1. All-out effort and commitment during your initial sprint through the MetaShred Diet.

2. The adequate level of commitment needed to maintain your fat loss for the rest of your life.

As you work to maintain your weight, you need to continue with similar—though less-intense—diet and fitness strategies. Unfortunately, due to the constant streams of environmental and social pressures on you each day to eat more and move less, maintaining your new body will be a constant uphill battle.

During the MetaShred Diet, you will abstain from alcohol. But afterward, you may be able to have five beers per week, while still maintaining your new body weight. That's great.

During the MetaShred Diet, you'll be 100 percent committed to the program. But afterward, you might just phone it in on Friday nights and all day Saturday—otherwise sticking to the plan the rest of the week. This may lead to you gaining back a couple of pounds, but if that's a trade-off you're comfortable with, it works for me.

This chapter is about helping you translate what you do during the 28-day MetaShred Diet into the rest of your life. Hopefully, it will help you see that it isn't all or nothing. There's a continuum of your eating and exercise habits and your body weight that you will need to navigate. But make no mistake: You are in control of your weight. The power is in your hands, and with the advice that follows, you can make sure it stays that way.

## The Morning After

Imagine that it is the morning of Day 29 (or Day 57 if you do the diet twice). What are you going to do? Hopefully, the same thing you did on Day 28, except maybe you'll indulge in your favorite meal that you've been missing for the last 4 weeks. (In case you're wondering, cornbread and BBQ brisket, lightly sauced, would be my choice.) Don't go crazy. Don't eat two boxes of sugary breakfast cereal or an entire pizza.

You're now entering the world of enjoyment, not gluttony. Eating a meal that you consider *off* your diet isn't an open invitation to reenact your favorite episode of *Man vs. Food*. Aim for quality over quantity. That's the mind-set you want going forward.

We've already talked about the importance of a solid fat-loss culture in your social circle. When you're coming off your initial MetaShred sprint, this support becomes even more important.

The truth is that 28 days is a short enough period of time that—if you were dedicated enough—you could power through without any social support. But trying to maintain that momentum and drive for your entire life without a positive group around you is a tall order.

Again, we have good insights on how to stay motivated with social support from that group of Greek weight-loss maintainers discussed earlier. In a more recent study published in June 2016, researchers assessed the difference in perceived social support between maintainers and regainers.[2] This might surprise you, but weight regainers received more support compared to weight-maintainers. Specifically, from their families and in the areas of diet and exercise. But how they perceived their social support was different.

Weight-maintainers received support that was positive and encouraging, while weight-regainers received support that was perceived as instructive. No one likes to be told what to do. How the people around you are supporting your fat-loss maintenance efforts matters more than the amount of support you are getting. What's the difference between positive and instructive support?

In this study, the family members of weight-maintainers would compliment the person's healthy eating habits while also eating healthy foods with them. Contrast this to the family members of weight-regainers. These folks would remind the regainers not to eat unhealthy or high-fat foods, while telling them to eat more healthy foods. Nobody likes a nag.

What happens in your social circles? As you transition away from your initial MetaShred Diet sprint, it will be important to audit the type of support that you're getting to see how it is influencing your progress.

## How to Monitor Your Body

I'm a big fan of the good old scale. Research shows that people who weigh themselves more often are more successful at maintaining their body weights.[3] I do have a fair number of clients who are totally averse to stepping on the scale, as it becomes a point of obsession for them. I respect this, and I don't insist that they weigh themselves every day. But I do insist that they find another barometer for assessing the overall state of their body size.

Is there a particular pair of jeans that fit really well? Perfect. Put those jeans on every week, and take note of how they fit. If they're starting to get a little snug, then that's a good signal that you need to audit your eating behaviors before things progress too far in the wrong direction.

If you aren't averse to the scale, just step on it every day when you wake up in the morning, after you go to the bathroom. Write down your weight, and then forget about it. Every 1 to 2 weeks, look at your list of body weights over the past several weeks, and take note of any trends that you see.

I use a Wi-Fi scale that automatically logs and graphs my body weight. I step on, step off, and don't think about it until Sunday evening when I review my weights for the week. You don't have to go high-tech like this, of course—a regular scale with a notepad and pencil works just as well.

The keys are measurement consistency—again, every morning when you wake up, right after you go to the bathroom—and perspective, so that you're reviewing 1 to 2 weeks of numbers at a time and not focused on a daily number. Your scale weight is a great tool for monitoring longer-term shifts in your body weight, but it's a terrible measure of day-to-day changes. The physiological measurement noise of water balance in your body is just too great over a 24-hour period. If you start fussing over why you were up 2 pounds yesterday but down 3 pounds today, you'll go mad.

## 3 Steps to a MetaShred Lifestyle

As you progress away from your first 100 percent focused MetaShred Diet sprint, you have a lot of resources available for making a successful transition to a MetaShred life-style. The difference is that you'll slowly increase your calories to the highest level that allows you to *maintain* your new weight. In fact, whenever I work with a client to transition out of a diet phase, the goal is always to significantly increase their calories without an appreciable increase in body fat.

## Step 1: Maintain Your New Body Weight and Diet

The first thing that people want to do when they get to the end of a diet is to start eating more. Slow down. The best thing you can do is to continue eating the same as you have been for another 1 to 2 weeks. Sure, you can enjoy a couple of meals that you've been missing or have a couple of drinks with friends, but for the most part, stay the course with what you've been doing. The longer you can stabilize your new body weight, the easier it will be to maintain that weight.

## Step 2: Increase Calories

You can increase your calories in one of two ways.

### 1. Change MetaDiet Levels

The first way is to move up one MetaDiet Level from the one that you're currently on. Let's say that you finished your 28 days of MetaShred Diet on MetaDiet Level C. You'll then move up to the phase 1 version of MetaDiet Level D, and follow it per the script. You can continue on Level D as long as you like; or, if your weight is stable—and you find yourself hungry—move up to MetaDiet Level E after 2 to 3 weeks.

### 2. Move Up the Hierarchy of Carbohydrates

Aside from changing MetaDiet Levels, the other way that you can transition off of your MetaShred Diet sprint is to move up the hierarchy of carbohydrates (see page 47). Essentially, you just add more whole grain/starch-based carbohydrates to your diet. This is a little slower, but more carb-centric approach. You would add these carbohydrates to the meal after your workout; or, on days that you don't work out, you have them at breakfast or dinner.

Breakfast is the preference for adding the starches on nonworkout days. That's because your liver sugar stores are low in the morning and you'll have all day to burn those carbs off. However, if you're a nighttime snacker, or find that your stress levels are particularly higher at night, adding these extra carbs to your dinner is a good option. Eating a larger-carbohydrate meal at night has been shown to provide greater satiety and, in one study, increased weight loss.[4] This might be because, when people are given more carbohydrates at night, they're less likely to snack on carbohydrate-based foods after dinner.

Here's what to add (pick one):

- ¼ pound raw potato
- 1 medium yam
- ½ cup cooked brown rice
- ¼ cup dry rolled oats
- 3 cups popped popcorn
- 1 thick slice wheat bread
- ½ cup cooked whole wheat pasta
- 2 corn tortillas

Any one of these is considered a portion of grain/starch that you can add to a meal. After 2 weeks, feel free to add another, and then another 2 weeks after that.

## Step 3: Keep Your Activity High

Because of the effects of exercise on how your body handles and processes carbohydrates, it's important to keep your exercise levels as high as you can.

## Find Your New "Why"

When you come to the end of your 28 or 56 days on the MetaShred Diet, you'll ask yourself, "Now what?"

This is an extremely common response once people lose all of the weight that they set out to drop. For most people, diet and exercise are always framed around fat loss. You've been eating and exercising certain ways for so many years as a means of losing weight.

Now that you've lost the weight, how should you eat and exercise? Why are you even doing it?

You need a new reason why. For the longest time, if you wanted to achieve a goal that was fitness related, your choices were a bodybuilding contest or a marathon. (Again with the extremes!) Fortunately, these days there are a lot of options for fitness challenges you can work toward and train for. From Tough Mudder to the Spartan Race to a GoRuck Light or Challenge (my personal favorite), there are many different kinds of events from which to choose. These can range from a simple 5-K to multiple-day races to a bicycling tour to a weight lifting competition. Groups of local CrossFit boxes frequently host fitness-based competitions to raise money for charity. Get involved and get after it.

You made a commitment to the MetaShred Diet, and you gave it your all. As a result, you've hopefully lost more fat than ever before and achieved your goals. Ride the wave of this commitment and pick your next challenge. What's your next mountain to conquer? Maybe it's even a specific mountain. (The Presidential Traverse in the White Mountains of New Hampshire is on my list.)

What's your next big personal challenge?

# Appendix: MetaShred Workouts

A solid fat loss program is essential for maximizing the power of the MetaShred diet for all the reasons we talked about in Chapter 4. Exercise helps you burn more calories around the clock while also helping your eat more food and still get lean due to the added calorie deficiet created by working out. Proper metabolic fat loss training also helps your body maintain and maybe even build muscle while you are MetaShred dieting ensuring that you have that *look* you are going for when you reach your goal weight.

I have reached out to 2 of the top trainers in the country—Joe Dowdell and Bill Hartman—and have asked them to provide you with fat loss training programs that will work with the MetaShred diet to enhance your ability to burn fat and get lean. Each workout of the workouts are unique so read through each of the workouts and their descriptions to before picking the one that is best for you.

Work hard, burn calories, and get MetaShredded.

# METASHRED MOVIE STAR FIT

## BY JOE DOWDELL

Joe Dowdell has spent more than 2 decades as the go to trainer in NYC for movie stars, models, and athletes that want to get in the best shape of their life. I was fortunate enough to work with Joe and many of his clients as the nutrition director of his gym in Manhattan for 5 years. During this time I saw Joe use his signature resistance training-cardio hybrid system to melt fat off his clients on command. With Joe's methods, you pair two resistance training exercises together but instead of resting after that pairing is complete, you add 30-60 seconds of a high intensity cardio movement. Adding the cardio components after every pair sets of your resistance training significantly increases the overall metabolic burn of the workout as you will clock in an extra nine high intensity cardio intervals by the time your workout is done. This is like adding an extra interval training workout inside your weight training workout!

## 2-Week Training Schedule

Monday: Program A
Tuesday: Interval Cardio Workout
Wednesday: Program B
Thursday: Interval Cardio Workout
Friday: Program A
Saturday: Low Intensity Cardio Workout
Sunday: Rest

Monday: Program B
Tuesday: Interval Cardio Workout
Wednesday: Program A
Thursday: Interval Cardio Workout
Friday: Program B
Saturday: Low Intensity Cardio Workout
Sunday: Rest

Repeat this 2-week cycle one
more time for a total of 4 weeks of
MetaShred Movie Star Fit

## PROGRAM A

| SEQ. | STRENGTH TRAINING | SETS | REPS | TEMPO | REST INTERVAL |
|------|-------------------|------|------|-------|---------------|
| A1 | **Barbell Front Squat** | 3-4* | 10-12 | 3010 | 30 sec. |
| A2 | **Flat Dumbbell Bench Press** | 3-4* | 10-12 | 3010 | 30 sec. |
| A3 | Fan Bike or Skipping Rope | 3-4* | 30-60 sec. | Fast | 90 sec. |
| B1 | **KB Swing** | 3-4* | 10-12 | 3010 | 30 sec. |
| B2 | **Single-Arm Dumbbell Row** | 3-4* | 10-12/side | 3010 | 30 sec. |
| B3 | Fan Bike or Skipping Rope | 3-4* | 30-60 sec. | Fast | 90 sec. |
| C1 | **Decline EZ-Bar Triceps Extension** | 3-4* | 10-12 | 3010 | 30 sec. |
| C2 | **Cable Core Press** | 3-4* | 30 sec./side | Hold | 30 sec. |
| C3 | Fan Bike or Skipping Rope | 3-4* | 30-60 sec. | Fast | 90 sec. |

*Number of sets in Weeks 3 & 4

**Week 1:** Perform 3 sets of each movement; rest 30 seconds between each exercise in the mini-circuit (eg. A1, A2, A3) and up to 90 seconds (or until your heart rate is at 60-65% of your Max HR whichever comes first) after the each mini-circuit.

**Week 2:** Perform 3 sets of each movement; rest 30 seconds between each exercise in the mini-circuit and up to 90 seconds (or until your heart rate is at 60-65% of your Max HR whichever comes first) after the each mini-circuit.

**Week 3:** Perform 4 sets of each movement; rest 30 seconds between each exercise in the mini-circuit and up to 90 seconds (or until your heart rate is at 60-65% of your Max HR whichever comes first) after the each mini-circuit.

**Week 4:** Perform 4 sets of each movement; rest 30 seconds between each exercise in the mini-circuit and up to 90 seconds (or until your heart rate is at 60-65% of your Max HR whichever comes first) after the each mini-circuit.

With A3, B3 & C3, if you can't do 60 seconds of work, start with 30 seconds and slowly increase to 60 seconds over the course of 6 weeks (i.e., 30 seconds in weeks 1 & 2; 45 seconds in weeks 3 & 4 and 60 seconds in weeks 5 & 6)

## A1 Barbell front squat

Hold a bar next to your chest with a shoulder-width, overhand grip. Raise your upper arms until they're parallel to the floor, letting the bar roll back so that it's resting on the front of your shoulders [A]. Push your hips back, bend your knees, and lower your body until the tops of your thighs are at least parallel to the floor [B]. Pause, and return to the starting position.

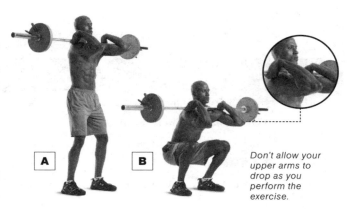

**A** **B**

*Don't allow your upper arms to drop as you perform the exercise.*

## A2 Flat dumbbell bench press

Grab a pair of dumbbells and lie on your back on a flat bench. Hold the dumbbells, palms facing forward, over your chest so they're nearly touching. Without changing the angle of your hands, lower the dumbbells to the sides of your chest. Pause, and press the weights back to the starting position as quickly as you can.

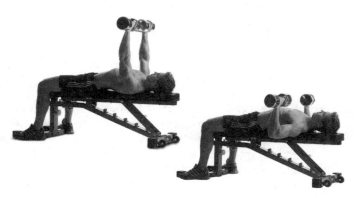

## B1 Kettlebell swing

Without rounding your lower back, push your hips back and swing a kettlebell between your legs. Thrust your hips forward and let the weight swing to shoulder level. Start the clock, do 10 swings, and rest; when you hit the 60-second mark, repeat.

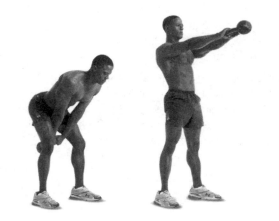

## B2 Single-arm dumbbell row

Hold a dumbbell in your right hand, and place your left hand and left knee on a flat bench. Lower your torso until it's almost parallel to the floor. Let the dumbbell hang at arm's length from your shoulder. Pull the dumbbell to the side of your chest. Pause, and return to the starting position. Do all reps, switch sides, and repeat.

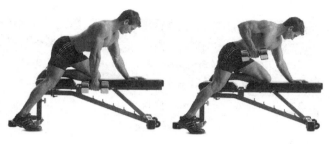

## 2B Decline EZ-bar triceps extension

Grab an EZ-curl bar using an over-hand grip, your hands a little less than shoulder-width apart. Lie faceup on a decline bench with your arms straight and hold the bar over your forehead. Without moving your upper arms, bend your elbows to lower the bar toward your head. Pause, and lift the weight back up by straightening your arms.

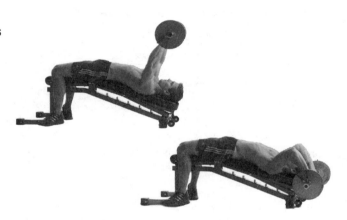

## C2 Cable core press

Attach a stirrup handle to the middle pulley of a cable station. With the cable taut, hold the handle against your chest with both hands and stand with your right side facing the stack **[A]**. Slowly press your arms forward until they're completely straight **[B]**. Pause for 5 seconds, and reverse the movement. Do all your reps, and then turn around and work your other side.

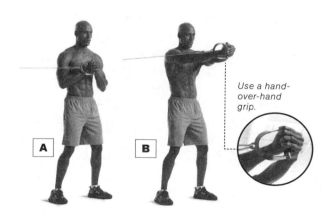

*Use a hand-over-hand grip.*

## PROGRAM B

| SEQ. | STRENGTH TRAINING | SETS | REPS | TEMPO | REST INTERVAL |
|------|-------------------|------|------|-------|---------------|
| A1 | **Dumbbell Bulgarian Split Squat** | 3-4* | 10-12/side | 2010 | 30 sec. |
| A2 | **Chinup (band assisted if necessary)** | 3-4* | 10-12 | 3010 | 30 sec. |
| A3 | Fan Bike or Skipping Rope | 3-4* | 30-60 sec. | Fast | 90 sec. |
| B1 | **Barbell Straight-Leg Deadlift** | 3-4* | 10-12 | 3010 | 30 sec. |
| B2 | **Incline Barbell Bench Press** | 3-4* | 10-12 | 3010 | 30 sec. |
| B3 | Fan Bike or Skipping Rope | 3-4* | 30-60 sec. | Fast | 90 sec. |
| C1 | **Seated Dumbbell Curl-to-Press** | 3-4* | 10-12 | 2020 | 30 sec. |
| C2 | **Barbell Rollout** | 3-4* | Up to 12 | 2020 | 30 sec. |
| C3 | Fan Bike or Skipping Rope | 3-4* | 30-60 sec. | Fast | 90 sec. |

*Number of sets in Weeks 3 & 4

**Week 1:** Perform 3 sets of each movement; rest 30 seconds between each exercise in the mini-circuit (eg. A1, A2, A3) and up to 90 seconds (or until your heart rate is at 60-65% of your Max HR whichever comes first) after the each mini-circuit.

**Week 2:** Perform 3 sets of each movement; rest 30 seconds between each exercise in the mini-circuit and up to 90 seconds (or until your heart rate is at 60-65% of your Max HR whichever comes first) after the each mini-circuit.

**Week 3:** Perform 4 sets of each movement; rest 30 seconds between each exercise in the mini-circuit and up to 90 seconds (or until your heart rate is at 60-65% of your Max HR whichever comes first) after the each mini-circuit.

**Week 4:** Perform 4 sets of each movement; rest 30 seconds between each exercise in the mini-circuit and up to 90 seconds (or until your heart rate is at 60-65% of your Max HR whichever comes first) after the each mini-circuit.

With A3, B3 & C3, if you can't do 60 seconds of work, start with 30 seconds and slowly increase to 60 seconds over the course of 6 weeks (i.e., 30 seconds in weeks 1 & 2; 45 seconds in weeks 3 & 4 and 60 seconds in weeks 5 & 6)

## A1 Dumbbell Bulgarian split squat

Hold a pair of dumbbells at arm's length, your palms facing each other. Stand in a staggered stance and place the top of your back foot on a bench. Lower your body as far as you can. Pause, and push back to the starting position. Do all reps, and then switch legs and repeat.

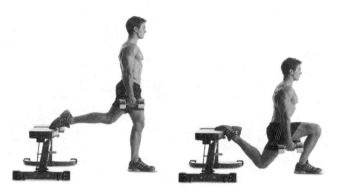

## A2 Chinup

Grab a chinup bar with a shoulder-width, underhand grip, and hang at arm's length **[A]**. Now squeeze your shoulder blades down and back, bend your elbows, and pull the top of your chest to the bar **[B]**. Pause, slowly lower your body back to the starting position, and repeat.

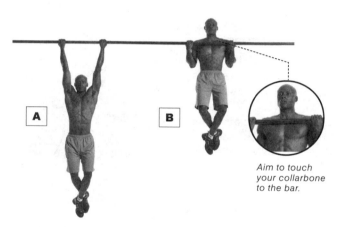

*Aim to touch your collarbone to the bar.*

## B1 Barbell straight-leg deadlift

Hold a barbell at arm's length using an overhand grip that's just beyond shoulder width. Keeping your knees slightly bent, bend at your hips and lower your torso until it's almost parallel to the floor. Pause, and raise your torso back to the starting position.

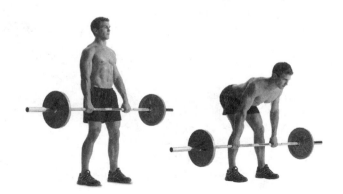

### B2 Incline barbell bench press

Set an adjustable bench to about 15 to 30 degrees. Lie faceup on the bench. With straight arms, hold a barbell using an overhand grip that's slightly beyond shoulder width. Lower the bar to your upper chest. Pause, and push the bar back up to the starting position.

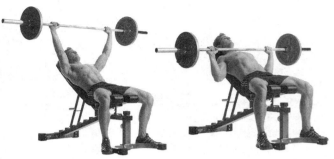

### C1 Seated dumbbell curl-to-press

Hold a pair of dumbbells at arm's length and sit on a bench. Without moving your upper arms, curl the dumbbells up to your shoulders. Rotate your palms so they face away from your body, and press the weights above your head. Return to the starting position and repeat.

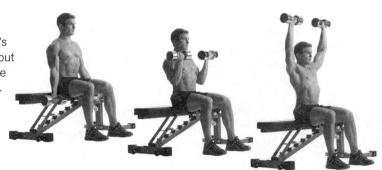

### C2 Barbell rollout

Load a barbell with 10-pound plates and affix collars. Kneel on the floor and grab the bar with an overhand, shoulder-width grip. Position your shoulders directly over the barbell and keep your lower back naturally arched [A]. Slowly roll the bar forward, extending your body as far as you can without letting your hips sag [B]. Pause for 2 seconds, and reverse the move to return to the starting position.

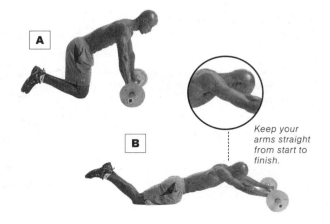

Keep your arms straight from start to finish.

# METASHRED LEAN EFFECTS
## BY BILL HARTMAN

Bill Hartman is a strength coach, physical therapist, and longtime advisor for *Men's Health*. Bill used the MetaShred Diet combined with his Lean Effects fat loss workouts to drop +30lbs leading up to his 50th birthday and as a result landed himself and his transformation a feature in *Men's Health* magazine. The MetaShred Lean Effects workouts are unique as they allow you to do more or less work during each training session based on how your body is feeling and functioning that day.

Here's how it works using the first workout as an example.

### Barbell Bench Press
3-6 sets x 6 reps
2 min. rest

You will see for the first exercise, barbell bench press, that there is a range of 3-6 sets. Sufficiently warm up on the bench press until you reach a weight where you can do 6 reps (and maybe a 7th if you really pushed). Rest for 2 minutes. Repeat your bench press efforts with the same weight for 6 reps. If after the 3rd set you can no longer get 6 quality reps at that preselected weight you are done with the bench press for the day.

On a day that you feel really fresh you might be able to get all 6 sets but on a day that you are tired and stressed your body might only be able to complete 4 sets. That is fine. Listening to your body in this way is called autoregulation. It is Jedi-level weight training.

For the next circuit in the workout, Bill provides ranges for both reps and rounds of the exercise groupings. The same autoregulation process applies here again.

## A. Dumbbell Bench Press x 8-10

75 seconds rest

## B. Offset Dumbbell Reverse Lunge x 8-10

75 seconds rest

## C. Face Pull x 8-10

75 seconds rest
Repeat 2-4 rounds

For each exercise, warm up until you get to a point where you can complete 10 repetitions of each movement. Rest 75 seconds between exercises. When you get to the end of the circuit, rest 75 seconds and repeat the circuit. If you are not able to complete the minimum number of quality reps (8 reps in this case) for any given exercise, that exercise gets dropped from the circuit and you complete the circuit with the remaining exercises.

Here's how it could look with the above circuit.

### Round 1

- Dumbbell Bench Press, 10 reps @ 80lbs
- rest 75 seconds
- Offset Dumbbell Reverse Lunge, 10 reps @ 45lbs
- rest 75 seconds
- Face Pull, 10 reps @ 35lbs
- rest 75 seconds

### Round 2

- Dumbbell Bench Press, 8 reps @ 80lbs
- rest 75 seconds
- Offset Dumbbell Reverse Lunge, 10 reps @ 45lbs
- rest 75 seconds
- Face Pull, 10 reps @ 35lbs
- rest 75 seconds

### Round 3

- Dumbbell Bench Press, 7 reps @ 80lbs
- rest 75 seconds
- Offset Dumbbell Reverse Lunge, 9 reps @ 45lbs
- rest 75 seconds
- Face Pull, 10 reps @ 35lbs
- rest 75 seconds

### Round 4

- Offset Dumbbell Reverse Lunge, 8 reps @ 45lbs
- rest 75 seconds
- Face Pull, 8 reps @ 35lbs
- rest 75 seconds

You can see that during the 3rd round of the circuit, the minimum target reps was not reached for the Dumbbell Bench Press so during the 4th round, that exercise was dropped from the circuit.

MetaShred Lean Effects training is great if you find that you are under a lot of stress or have dips in energy during the week as it allows you to get in the fat loss training your body needs to get lean while also working with your body to do this and not against it. Maybe after 4 weeks of MetaShred Lean Effects training, you'll be ready for your own magazine feature!

# Week 1

| DAY 1 | DAY 2 | DAY 3 | DAY 4 | DAY 5 |
|---|---|---|---|---|
| Dynamic Warm-up<br><br>**1. BB Bench Press**<br>3-6 sets x 6 reps<br>2 min. rest<br><br>**2A. DB Bench Press x 8-10**<br>75 sec. rest<br><br>**2B. Offset DB Reverse Lunge x 8-10**<br>75 sec. rest<br><br>**2C. Face Pull x 8-10**<br>75 sec. rest<br>Repeat 2-4 rounds<br><br>**3. BB Rollout**<br>2-3 x hold for 5 breaths<br>60 sec. rest | 45-60 minutes of continuous activity where you can barely maintain a conversation | Dynamic Warm-up<br><br>**1. Chinup**<br>3-6 sets x 4<br>2 min. rest<br><br>**2A. One-Arm Lat Pulldown x 10-12**<br>75 sec. rest<br><br>**2B. Front Squat x 10-12**<br>75 sec. rest<br><br>**2C. Seated DB Curl-to-Press x 10-12**<br>75 sec. rest<br>Repeat 2-4 rounds<br><br>**3. Half-Kneeling Cable Chop**<br>2-3 x 12<br>60 sec. rest | 45-60 minutes of continuous activity where you can barely maintain a conversation | Dynamic Warm-up<br><br>**1. Deadlift**<br>3-6 sets x 5<br>2-3 min. rest<br><br>**2A. Single-Arm DB Row x 6-8**<br>75 sec. rest<br><br>**2B. Explosive Pushup**<br>x 6-8<br>75 sec. rest<br><br>**2C. DB Stepup x 6-8**<br>75 sec. rest<br>Repeat 2-4 rounds<br><br>**3. Cable Core Press**<br>2-3 x 30 sec. each side<br>60 sec. rest |

# Week 2

| DAY 1 | DAY 2 | DAY 3 | DAY 4 | DAY 5 |
|---|---|---|---|---|
| Dynamic Warm-up<br><br>**1. BB Bench Press**<br>3-6 sets x 5<br>2 min. rest<br><br>**2A. DB Bench Press x 6-8**<br>60 sec. rest<br><br>**2B. Offset DB Reverse Lunge x 6-8**<br>60 sec. rest<br><br>**2C. Face Pull x 6-8**<br>60 sec. rest<br>Repeat 2-4 rounds<br><br>**3. BB Rollout**<br>2-3 x hold for 5 breaths<br>60 sec. rest | 45-60 minutes of continuous activity where you can barely maintain a conversation | Dynamic Warm-up<br><br>**1. Chinup**<br>3-6 sets x 6<br>2 min. rest<br><br>**2A. One-Arm Lat Pulldown x 8-10**<br>60 sec. rest<br><br>**2B. Front Squat x 8-10**<br>60 sec. rest<br><br>**2C. Seated DB Curl-to-Press x 8-10**<br>60 sec. rest<br>Repeat 2-4 rounds<br><br>**3. Half-Kneeling Cable Chop**<br>2-3 x 12<br>60 sec. rest | 45-60 minutes of continuous activity where you can barely maintain a conversation | Dynamic Warm-up<br><br>**1. Deadlift**<br>3-6 sets x 4<br>2 min. rest<br><br>**2A. Single-Arm DB Row x 10-12**<br>60 sec. rest<br><br>**2B. Pushup**<br>x 10-12<br>60 sec. rest<br><br>**2C. DB Stepup x 10-12**<br>2 min. rest<br>Repeat 2-4 rounds<br><br>**3. Cable Core Press**<br>2-3 x 30 sec.<br>60 sec. rest |

# Week 3

| DAY 1 | DAY 2 | DAY 3 | DAY 4 | DAY 5 |
|---|---|---|---|---|
| Dynamic Warm-up | 45-60 minutes of continuous activity where you can barely maintain a conversation | Dynamic Warm-up | 45-60 minutes of continuous activity where you can barely maintain a conversation | Dynamic Warm-up |
| **1. BB Bench Press** 3-6 sets x 4 2 min. rest | | **1. Chinup** 3-6 sets x 5 2 min. rest | | **1. Deadlift** 3-6 sets x 6 2 min. rest |
| **2A. DB Bench Press x 10-12** 45 sec. rest | | **2A. Single-Arm Lat Pulldown x 6-8** 45 sec. rest | | **2A. Single-Arm DB Row x 8-10** 45 sec. rest |
| **2B. Offset DB Reverse Lunge x 10-12** 45 sec. rest | | **2B. Front Squat x 6-8** 45 sec. rest | | **2B. Tempo Pushup x 8-10** 45 sec. rest |
| **2C. Face Pull x 10-12** 45 sec. rest Repeat until drop-off | | **2C. Seated DB Curl-to-Press x 6-8** 45 sec. rest Repeat until drop-off | | **2C. DB Stepup x 8-10** 2 min. rest Repeat 2-4 rounds |
| **3. BB Rollout** 2-3 x hold for 5 breaths 60 sec. rest | | **3. Half-Kneeling Cable Chop** 2-3 x 12 60 sec. rest | | **3. Cable Core Press** 2-3 x 30 sec. 60 sec. rest |

# Week 4

| DAY 1 | DAY 2 | DAY 3 | DAY 4 | DAY 5 |
|---|---|---|---|---|
| Dynamic Warm-up | 45-60 minutes of continuous activity where you can barely maintain a conversation | Dynamic Warm-up | 45-60 minutes of continuous activity where you can barely maintain a conversation | Dynamic Warm-up |
| **1. BB Bench Press** 2 sets x 4 2 min. rest | | **1. Chinup** 2 sets x 4 2 min. rest | | **1. Deadlift** 2 sets x 4 2 min. rest |
| **2A. DB Bench Press x 15** 30 sec. rest | | **2A. Single-Arm Lat Pulldown x 15** 30 sec. rest | | **2A. Single-Arm DB Row x 15** 30 sec. rest |
| **2B. Offset DB Reverse Lunge x 15** 30 sec. rest | | **2B. Front Squat x 15** 30 sec. rest | | **2B. Pushup x 15** 30 sec. rest |
| **2C. Face Pull x 15** 30 sec. rest Repeat 2-4 rounds | | **2C. Seated DB Curl-to-Press x 15** 30 sec. rest Repeat 2-4 rounds | | **2C. DB Stepup x 15 each side** 30 sec. rest Repeat 2-4 rounds |
| **3. BB Rollout** 2 x hold for 5 breaths 60 sec. rest | | **3. Half-Kneeling Cable Chop** 2 x 12 60 sec. rest | | **3. Cable Core Press** 2 x 30 sec. 60 sec. rest |

## 1 Barbell bench press

Grab a barbell and lie on a bench. Using an overhand grip that's just beyond shoulder width, hold the bar above your sternum, keeping your arms straight. Lower the bar to your chest, and then push it back to the starting position.

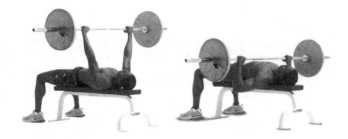

## 2A Dumbbell bench press

Grab a pair of dumbbells and lie on your back on a flat bench. Hold the dumbbells, palms facing forward, over your chest so they're nearly touching. Without changing the angle of your hands, lower the dumbbells to the sides of your chest. Pause, and press the weights back to the starting position as quickly as you can.

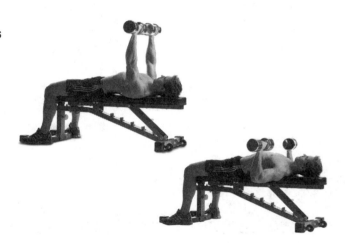

## 2B Offset dumbbell reverse lunge

Stand holding a dumbbell in your right hand next to your shoulder, with your arm bent [A]. With your left foot, step backward into a reverse lunge and lower your body until your back knee almost touches the floor [B]. Push yourself back to the starting position and repeat. Do all your reps, and then switch arms and lunge backward with your right leg.

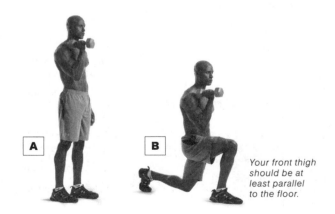

*Your front thigh should be at least parallel to the floor.*

## 2C Face pull

Attach a rope to the high pulley of a cable station. Grab the ends of the rope with your palms facing each other. Starting with your arms straight, pull the middle of the rope toward your nose (flare your elbows). Pause, and repeat.

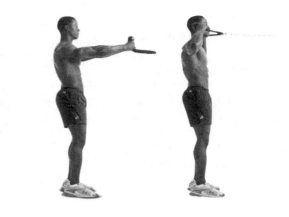

## 3 Barbell rollout

Load a barbell with 10-pound plates and affix collars. Kneel on the floor and grab the bar with an overhand, shoulder-width grip. Position your shoulders directly over the barbell and keep your lower back naturally arched **[A]**. Slowly roll the bar forward, extending your body as far as you can without letting your hips sag **[B]**. Pause for 2 seconds, and reverse the move to return to the starting position.

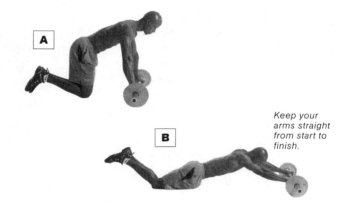

*Keep your arms straight from start to finish.*

## 1 Chinup

Grab a chinup bar with a shoulder-width, underhand grip, and hang at arm's length **[A]**. Now squeeze your shoulder blades down and back, bend your elbows, and pull the top of your chest to the bar **[B]**. Pause, slowly lower your body back to the starting position, and repeat.

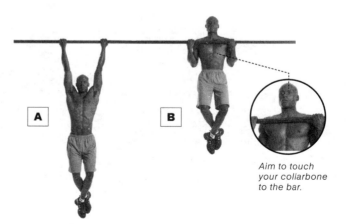

*Aim to touch your collarbone to the bar.*

### 2A Single-arm lat pulldown

Attach a handle to the high pulley of a cable station. Grab the handle with one hand and sit in front of the weight stack. Without rotating your torso, pull the handle to the side of your chest. Do all your reps, switch hands, and repeat.

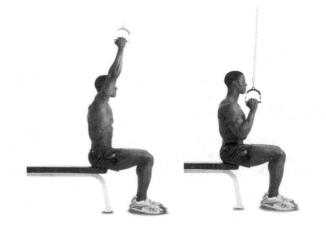

### 2B Barbell front squat

Hold a bar next to your chest with a shoulder-width, overhand grip. Raise your upper arms until they're parallel to the floor, letting the bar roll back so that it's resting on the front of your shoulders **[A]**. Push your hips back, bend your knees, and lower your body until the tops of your thighs are at least parallel to the floor **[B]**. Pause, and return to the starting position.

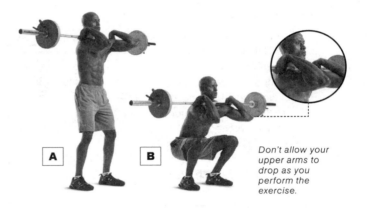

A   B

*Don't allow your upper arms to drop as you perform the exercise.*

### 2C Seated dumbbell curl-to-press

Hold a pair of dumbbells at arm's length and sit on a bench. Without moving your upper arms, curl the dumbbells up to your shoulders. Rotate your palms so they face away from your body, and press the weights above your head. Return to the starting position and repeat.

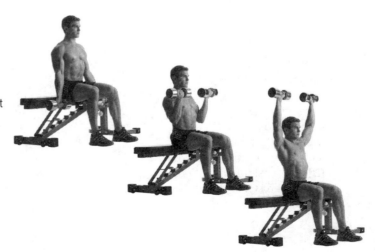

### 3 Half-kneeling cable chop

Attach a rope handle to the high pulley of a cable station. With your left side to the stack, kneel as shown. Grab the rope with both hands above shoulder height. Trying not to move your torso, pull the rope past your right hip. Reverse the move. Do all your reps, turn, and repeat on your other side. That's 1 set.

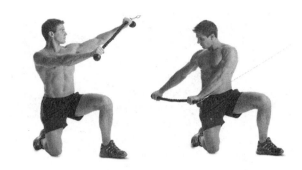

### 1 Barbell deadlift

Load a barbell and roll it against your shins. Bend at your hips and knees and grab the bar using an overhand grip. Without rounding your lower back, stand up. Then lower the barbell back to the floor, keeping it as close to your body as possible.

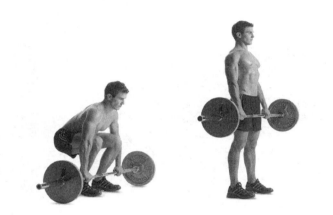

### 2A Single-arm dumbbell row

Hold a dumbbell in your right hand, and place your left hand and left knee on a flat bench. Lower your torso until it's almost parallel to the floor. Let the dumbbell hang at arm's length from your shoulder. Pull the dumbbell to the side of your chest. Pause, and return to the starting position. Do all reps, switch sides, and repeat.

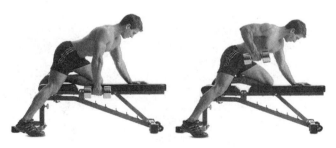

### 2B Explosive pushup

Assume a pushup position. Your body should form a straight line from your head to your ankles. Bend your elbows and lower your body until your chest nearly touches the floor. Then push up with enough force for your hands to come off the floor. Land and repeat.

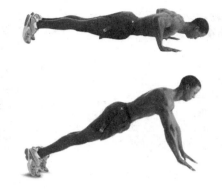

### 2C Dumbbell stepup

Grab a pair of dumbbells and place your right foot on a box or step. Push through your right heel until your right leg is straight. Lower yourself back down. Do all your reps with your right leg, and repeat with your left.

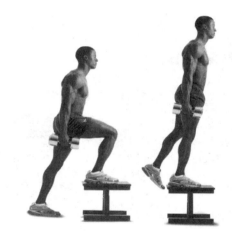

### 3 Cable core press

Attach a stirrup handle to the middle pulley of a cable station. With the cable taut, hold the handle against your chest with both hands and stand with your right side facing the stack [A]. Slowly press your arms forward until they're completely straight [B]. Pause for 5 seconds, and reverse the movement. Do all your reps, and then turn around and work your other side.

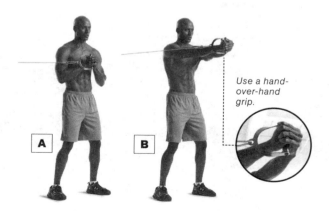

Use a hand-over-hand grip.

# Endnotes

## Chapter 1

1   J. A. Linde et al., "Weight Loss Goals and Treatment Outcomes Among Overweight Men and Women Enrolled in a Weight Loss Trial," *International Journal of Obesity* 29, no. 8 (August 2015): 1002-5.

2   Farlyle Northwehr and J. Yang, "Goal Setting Frequency and Use of Behavioral Strategies Related to Diet and Physical Activity," *Health Education Research* 22, no. 4 (August 2007): 532-38.

## Chapter 2

1   "Very Low-Calorie Diets," National Institute of Diabetes and Digestive and Kidney Diseases, https://www.niddk.nih.gov/health-information/health-topics/weight-control/very-low-calorie-diets/Pages/very-low-calorie-diets.aspx (accessed September 23, 2016).

2   Jesse Itzler, *Living with a SEAL: 31 Days Training with the Toughest Man on the Planet* (New York: Center Street, 2015).

## Chapter 3

1   Klaas R Westerterp, "Diet Induced Thermogenesis," *Nutrition & Metabolism* 1 (2004): 5.

2   Klaas R.Westerterp, "Long Term Effect of Physical Activity on Energy Balance and Body Composition," *British Journal of Nutrition* 68 (1992): 21-30.

3   Richard P. Feynman, "Cargo Cult Science," Caltech, http://calteches.library.caltech.edu/51/2/CargoCult.htm (accessed September 23, 2016).

4   A. M. Harris, M. D. Jensen, and J. A. Levine, "Weekly Changes in Basal Metabolic Rate with Eight Weeks of Overfeeding," *Obesity* 14, no. 4 (April 2006): 690-95.

5   A. M. Joosen, A. H. Bakker, and K. R. Westerterp, "Metabolic Efficiency and Energy Expenditure during Short-Term Overfeeding," *Physiology & Behavior* 85, no. 5 (August 7, 2005): 593-97.

## Chapter 4

1   Food and Nutrition Board of the Institute of Medicine, *Dietary Reference Intakes: The Essential Guide to Nutrient Requirements* (Washington, DC: National Academies Press, 2006), 169.

2    https://www.nationalacademies.org/hmd/~/media/Files/Activity%20Files/Nutrition/DRIs/DRI_Macronutrients.pdf

3    P. Marckmann et al., "High-Protein Diets and Renal Health," *Journal of Renal Nutrition* 25, no. 1 (January 2015): 1–5.

4    M. R. Charlton, "Protein Metabolism and Liver Disease," *Baillière's Clinical Endocrinology and Metabolism* 10, no. 4 (October 1996): 617–35.

5    J. P. Bonjour, "Protein Intake and Bone Health," *International Journal for Vitamin and Nutrition Research* 81, nos. 2–3 (March 2011): 134–42.

6    Heather J. Leidy et al., "The Role of Protein in Weight Loss and Maintenance," *American Journal of Clinical Nutrition* 101, no. 6 (June 2015): S1320–S1329.

7    David S. Weigle et al., "A High-Protein Diet Induces Sustained Reductions in Appetite, Ad Libitum Caloric Intake, and Body Weight Despite Compensatory Changes in Diurnal Plasma Leptin and Ghrelin Concentrations," *American Journal of Clinical Nutrition* 82, no. 1 (July 2005): 41–48.

8    Heather J. Leidy et al., "Neural Responses to Visual Food Stimuli after a Normal vs. Higher Protein Breakfast in Breakfast-Skipping Teens: A Pilot fMRI Study," *Obesity* 19 (October 2011): 2019–25.

9    Jeff Goodell, "Steve Jobs: Rolling Stone's 2003 Interview," *Rolling Stone*, www.rollingstone.com/music/news/steve-jobs-rolling-stones-2003-interview-20111006 (accessed September 23, 2016).

10   Heather J. Leidy et al., "The Influence of Higher Protein Intake and Greater Eating Frequency on Appetite Control in Overweight and Obese Men," *Obesity* 18, no. 9 (September 2010): 1725–32.

11   University of Texas Medical Branch at Galveston, "Moderate Amounts of Protein per Meal Found Best for Building Muscle," ScienceDaily, October 27, 2009, https://www.sciencedaily.com/releases/2009/10/091026125543.htm.

12   Madonna M. Mamerow et al., "Dietary Protein Distribution Positively Influences 24-H Muscle Protein Synthesis in Healthy Adults," *Journal of Nutrition* 144, no. 6 (June 2014): 876–80.

13   J. Bohé et al., "Latency and Duration of Stimulation of Human Muscle Protein Synthesis during Continuous Infusion of Amino Acids," *Journal of Physiology* 532 (April 15, 2011): 575–79.

14   D. Paddon-Jones et al., "Exogenous Amino Acids Stimulate Human Muscle Anabolism without Interfering with the Response to Mixed Meal Ingestion," *American Journal of Physiology–Endocrinology and Metabolism* 288, no. 4 (2005): E761–67.

15   A. J. Nordmann et al., "Effects of Low-Carbohydrate vs Low-Fat Diets on Weight Loss and Cardiovascular Risk Factors: A Meta-Analysis of Randomized Controlled Trials," *Archives of Internal Medicine* 166, no. 3 (2006): 285–93.

16    David Baker and Natacha Keramidas, "The Psychology of Hunger," *Monitor on Psychology* 44, no. 9 (October 2013): 66.

17    R. W. Bryner et al., "Effects of Resistance vs. Aerobic Training Combined with an 800 Calorie Liquid Diet on Lean Body Mass and Resting Metabolic Rate," *Journal of the American College of Nutrition* 18, no. 2 (April 1999): 115-21.

## Chapter 5

1     Centers for Disease Control and Prevention, "1 in 3 Adults Don't Get Enough Sleep," news release, February 18, 2016, www.cdc.gov/media/releases/2016/p0215-enough-sleep.html.

2     National Sleep Foundation, "Lack of Sleep Is Affecting Americans, Finds the National Sleep Foundation," news release, December 2014, https://sleepfoundation.org/media-center/press-release/lack-sleep-affecting-americans-finds-the-national-sleep-foundation.

3     Sanjay R. Patel and Frank B. Hu, "Short Sleep Duration and Weight Gain: A Systematic Review," *Obesity* 16, no. 3 (March 2008): 643-53.

4     M. Sivak, "Sleeping More as a Way to Lose Weight," *Obesity Reviews* 7, no. 3 (August 2006): 295-96.

5     E. C. Hanlon et al., "Sleep Restriction Enhances the Daily Rhythm of Circulating Levels of Endocannabinoid 2-Arachidonoylglycerol," *Sleep* 39, no. 3 (March 2016): 653-64.

6     Josiane L. Broussard et al., "Elevated Ghrelin Predicts Food Intake during Experimental Sleep Restriction," *Obesity* 24, no. 1 (January 2016): 132-38.

7     R. H. Anderberg et al., "The Stomach-Derived Hormone Ghrelin Increases Impulsive Behavior," *Neuropsychopharmacology* 41, no. 5 (April 2016): 1199-1209.

8     S. M. Schmid et al., "A Single Night of Sleep Deprivation Increases Ghrelin Levels and Feelings of Hunger in Normal-Weight Healthy Men," *Journal of Sleep Research* 17, no. 3 (September 2008): 331-34.

9     K. Spiegel et al., "Brief Communication: Sleep Curtailment in Healthy Young Men Is Associated with Decreased Leptin Levels, Elevated Ghrelin Levels, and Increased Hunger and Appetite," *Annals of Internal Medicine* 141, no. 11 (December 7, 2004): 846-50.

10    M. N. Rao et al., "Subchronic Sleep Restriction Causes Tissue-Specific Insulin Resistance," *Journal of Clinical Endocrinology & Metabolism* 100, no. 4 (April 2015): 1664-71.

11    Sebastian M. Schmid et al., "Short-Term Sleep Loss Decreases Physical Activity under Free-Living Conditions but Does Not Increase Food Intake under Time-Deprived Laboratory Conditions in Healthy Men," *American Journal of Clinical Nutrition* 90, no. 6 (December 2009): 1476-82.

12   L. E. Bromley et al., "Sleep Restriction Decreases the Physical Activity of Adults at Risk for Type 2 Diabetes," *Sleep* 35, no. 7 (July 1, 2012): 977–84.

13   J. R. Cho et al., "Let There Be No Light: The Effect of Bedside Light on Sleep Quality and Background Electroencephalographic Rhythms," *Sleep Medicine* 14, no. 12 (December 2013): 1422–25.

14   R. Killick et al., "Metabolic and Hormonal Effects of 'Catch-Up' Sleep in Men with Chronic, Repetitive, Lifestyle-Driven Sleep Restriction," *Clinical Endocrinology* 83, no. 4 (October 2015): 498–507.

15   Arlet V. Nedeltcheva et al., "Insufficient Sleep Undermines Dietary Efforts to Reduce Adiposity," *Annals of Internal Medicine* 153, no. 7 (October 5, 2010): 435–41.

16   J. Kounios et al., "The Prepared Mind: Neural Activity Prior to Problem Presentation Predicts Subsequent Solution by Sudden Insight," *Psychological Science* 17 (October 2006): 882–90.

17   R. A. Krukowski et al., "Internet-Based Weight Control: The Relationship Between Web Features and Weight Loss," *Telemedicine Journal and e-Health* 14, no. 8 (2008): 775–82.

## Chapter 6

1   "Eat a Variety of Foods," Health.gov, https://health.gov/dietaryguidelines/dga95/variety.htm (accessed September 23, 2016).

2   C. D. Gardner et al., "Micronutrient Quality of Weight-Loss Diets That Focus on Macronutrients: Results from the A TO Z Study," *American Journal of Clinical Nutrition* 92, no. 2 (August 2010): 304–12.

3   F. H. Nielsen and H. C. Lukaski, "Update on the Relationship Between Magnesium and Exercise," *Magnesium Research* 19, no. 3 (2006): 180–9.

4   K. Tanabe et al., "Efficacy of Oral Magnesium Administration on Decreased Exercise Tolerance in a State of Chronic Sleep Deprivation," *Japanese Circulation Journal* 62 (1998): 341–46.

5   Micah J. Drummond and Blake B. Rasmussen, "Leucine-Enriched Nutrients and the Regulation of Mammalian Target of Rapamycin Signaling and Human Skeletal Muscle Protein Synthesis," *Current Opinion in Clinical Nutrition & Metabolic Care* 11, no. 3 (May 2008): 222–26.

6   D. Frankenfield, L. Roth-Yousey, and C. Compher, "Comparison of Predictive Equations for Resting Metabolic Rate in Healthy Nonobese and Obese Adults: A Systematic Review," *Journal of the American Dietetic Association* 105, no. 5 (May 2005): 775–89.

7   J. Boullata et al., "Accurate Determination of Energy Needs in Hospitalized Patients," *Journal of the American Dietetic Association* 107, no. 3 (March 2007): 393–401.

8    J. Arthur Harris and Francis G. Benedict, "A Biometric Study of Human Basal Metabolism," October 8, 1918, www.ncbi.nlm.nih.gov/pmc/articles/PMC1091498/pdf/pnas01945-0018.pdf (accessed September 23, 2016).

## Chapter 9

1    Julie E. Obbagy et al., "Chefs' Opinions about Reducing the Calorie Content of Menu Items in Restaurants," *Obesity* 19, no. 2 (2011): 332–37.

2    M. Condrasky et al., "Chef's Opinions of Restaurant Portion Sizes," *Obesity* 15 (2007): 2086–93.

3    L. S. Roe., J. S. Meengs, and B. J. Rolls, "Salad and Satiety: The Effect of Timing of Salad Consumption on Meal Energy Intake," *Appetite* 58, no. 1 (2012): 242–48.

## Chapter 10

1    E. Karfopoulou et al., "Behaviours Associated with Weight Loss Maintenance and Regaining in a Mediterranean Population Sample. A Qualitative Study," *Clinical Obesity* 3, no. 5 (October 2013): 141–49.

2    E. Karfopoulou et al., "The Role of Social Support in Weight Loss Maintenance: Results from the MedWeight Study," *Journal of Behavioral Medicine* 39, no. 3 (June 2016): 511–18.

3    Thomas, J. Graham et al., "Weight-Loss Maintenance for 10 Years in the National Weight Control Registry," *American Journal of Preventive Medicine* 46, no. 1 (2014): 17–23.

4    S. Sofer et al., "Greater Weight Loss and Hormonal Changes after 6 Months Diet with Carbohydrates Eaten Mostly at Dinner," *Obesity* 19, no. 10 (October 2011): 2006–14.

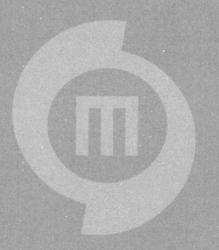

# Index

**Boldface** page references indicate photos. <u>Underscored</u> references indicate boxed text.